So, You Don't Want to Get CANCER?

A Research-Based Guide to the Lifestyle Changes
You Can Make to Prevent Cancer

Dr. David Ingram

So, You Don't Want to Get Cancer?

A Research-Based Guide to the Lifestyle Changes You Can Make to Prevent Cancer

Disclaimer

The information contained in this book is current at the time of this writing. Although all attempts have been made to verify the information provided in this publication, neither the author nor the publisher assumes any responsibility for errors, omissions, or contrary interpretations of the subject matter herein.

This book is for educational purposes only. The views expressed are those of the author and should not be taken as expert instruction or commands. The reader is responsible for his or her own actions. Neither the author nor the publisher assumes any responsibility or liability whatsoever on the behalf of the reader of these materials.

At times links might be used to illustrate a point, technique, or best practice. Readers should do their own research, make appropriate comparisons, and form their own decisions as to what is best for them.

The information, ideas, and techniques in this book are not medical advice or treatment, but rather knowledge intended to assist the reader. It is the responsibility of the reader to seek treatment for any medical, mental, or emotional conditions that might warrant professional care.

Artist: Alison Fennell, www.etsy.com/uk/shop/ThePotteringArtist

Editor: Joni Wilson

Layout and Design: Katharine Middleton, www.inkboxgraphics.com.au

Publisher: Ognid Publications

ISBN 9780648715108

Cancer and the Crab

Latin: cancer = crab

Greek: karkinos (carcinos) = crab

First used by the Greek physician,
Hippocrates (460-370 BC), to describe
an ulcer-forming tumor with arm-like
projections away from the central mass,
resembling a crab.

Also used in Astrology, where Cancer
is the 4th sign of the Zodiac, representing
the giant crab that attacked Heracles
in Greek mythology.

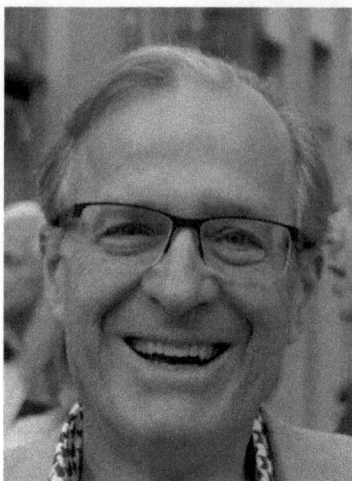

Author Profile

Dr. David Ingram is a specialist cancer surgeon. He has undertaken research investigating the relationship between diet, hormones, and other aspects of lifestyle and breast cancer, publishing more than eighty articles in scientific journals. He is a past associate professor of surgery at the University of Western Australia and is an avid follower of current medical literature on preventive aspects of cancer.

During his practice, he came to realize that most people do not know there is much they can do to prevent getting cancer. There is also a lot of misinformation. He saw a need to provide an evidence-based information resource, this book, for everyone who has an interest in looking after their health.

Dr. Ingram did his undergraduate medical studies at the University of Melbourne and has a postgraduate master's degree from the University of Western Australia. He lives in Perth, Western Australia.

More information about Dr. Ingram can be found on his website:
www.dontwantcancer.com.au

Contents

Author Profile   4
Preface   7

Part 1—The Basics

What Is Cancer?   10
The Cancer Problem   13
Genetics and Cancer   16
Finding the Cause   19
Understanding Cancer Research   22

Part 2—The Factors

Alcohol   26
Cell Phones   30
Chronic Infections   32
Coffee   36
Diet and Cancer   40
Excess Body Fat   52
The Gut Microbiome   59
Medications to Prevent Cancer   62
Pesticides and Herbicides   65
Physical Activity   67
Preventive Surgery   71
Radiation   74
Smoking   80
Stress and Cancer   84
Vitamins and Minerals   87

Part 3—The Common Cancers

Gastrointestinal Tract Cancers   98
     Cancer of the Oral Cavity   99
     Esophageal Cancer   101
     Gastric Cancer   105
     Colorectal Cancer   109
     Anal Cancer   117
Liver Cancer   118
Pancreatic Cancer   122

The Female Cancers
    Breast Cancer   125
    Ovarian Cancer   132
    Uterine Cancer   134
The Male Cancers
    Prostate Cancer   140
    Testicular Cancer   143
Cancers of the Respiratory Tract
    Nasopharyngeal Cancer   145
    Cancers of the Larynx, Bronchi, and Lung   147
    Mesothelioma   150
Cancers of the Urinary Tract
    Renal Cancer   152
    Bladder Cancer   154
Skin Cancer   156
Thyroid Cancer   166
Brain Tumors   167
Blood and Lymphatic Cancers   169
The Final Word   171
Glossary of Terms   173
Acknowledgments   177

Preface

As a cancer surgeon, I have spent most of my life caring for patients with cancer. The thing that has impressed me most about the people I have treated is their resilience in the face of adversity. But, despite the brave fronts, everyone is scarred. Not just the physical scarring from surgery but scarred emotionally. There is always the underlying anxiety: "Will the cancer return and kill me?" "Will I be around to see my family?" "Will I be disfigured by my treatment?" For some, these are just passing thoughts; others are never really free. The unfortunate thing is that sometimes it does come to pass—some people die from cancer.

It became clear to me that *treating* cancer is not the best approach. If we could *prevent* cancer from happening in the first place, then these anxieties would not be a problem. Furthermore, it would not be necessary to go through the surgery, chemotherapy, radiation therapy, and other procedures that are so often needed in cancer treatment. You might think that there is nothing you can do to stop getting cancer, but that is not true. It has been estimated that up to 40 percent of cancers are preventable. There are changes you can make that will significantly reduce your chances of getting this disease. Some are easy, but some require a lot of effort and willpower.

It used to be thought that we just had to find the right drug or vaccine, and we could prevent or even cure cancer. I have got to admit, that as a young researcher, I thought that I just needed to find out what it was in our diet that did the damage, remove it, and cancer would no longer be an issue. There were even conspiracy theories that the big drug companies could make the necessary drugs to prevent or cure cancer, but they wouldn't because they were making so much money making drugs to treat it. None of this is true. The cause of cancer is multifactorial, so there is no one prevention or cure.

This book is not about treating cancer. It is about what you can do in a practical way to reduce your chances of developing the disease in the first place, that is, preventing cancer. No one can guarantee that you will not get cancer at some stage in your life. The statistics are that more than one in three of us will get some form of cancer before we die, but there are things you can do to prevent cancer from ever happening. This is the ideal.

But if you never get cancer, was it because you did all the right things, or were you never destined to get it anyway? There's no way of knowing. In some ways, this makes it difficult. We work harder to achieve a goal if we know there is a reward at the end. In this situation, after years of hard work following all the preventive strategies, there is no reward, just wondering if it was all worthwhile. You would never know, but what a great situation to be in, never getting cancer!

I have not covered every cancer in this book. The rare cancers, such as sarcomas, are so uncommon that not a lot is known about why they occur, and so we cannot give a lot of advice about what to do so you do not get sarcoma. What I have principally concentrated on is the common cancers. The abdominal cancers—esophagus, stomach, liver, pancreas, colon, rectum, and anal cancers; the reproductive system cancers—breast, cervix, uterus, and ovary in women, and testicular and prostate cancer in men; skin and melanoma; the urinary cancers, such as kidney and bladder; and the big killer, lung cancer. These combined make up more than 80 percent of all cancer disease. Furthermore, these have been studied more extensively and we know more about why they occur, and so how they might be prevented.

My goal is to share with you what I've learned through many years of experience and research. I will provide information that gives you a background and a foundation to learn more details about understanding cancer. There are also "What You Should Do" summaries that give you specific ways to change your lifestyle. If you are determined you can decrease your chances of getting cancer.

Part I—The Basics

What Is Cancer?

The Cancer Problem

Genetics and Cancer

Finding the Cause

Understanding Cancer Research

What Is Cancer?

Cancer is a complex and varied disease. It can occur in any of the body's organs, and in any one organ it can take various forms. Furthermore, these forms can behave differently from person to person. For all this, the underlying process is basically the same: an uncontrolled growth of cells.

The body, consisting of billions of cells, has amazing control mechanisms that result in it functioning the way it does, so we thrive and reproduce and continue the species. These control mechanisms can become deranged, and in the case of cancer, this loss of control relates to cell growth.

Complex mechanisms determine when a cell multiplies (mitosis), how long it lives, and when it dies (apoptosis). This process of control of cell growth and death is determined by specific genes. If these particular genes are damaged and cannot be repaired, it is possible for cell multiplication to go on and on, with no control over cell death to balance the growth. This is the basic process of cancer.

How Does Cancer Start?

The genes that control cell growth are either oncogenes—these genes control when a cell needs to divide and form a new cell to replace an aging or damaged cell—or tumor suppressor genes that inhibit cell division when growth is not needed. Damage to an oncogene can result in what we call over-expression, where it works overtime to make cells divide and multiply. When there is damage to a tumor suppressor gene, there might be no inhibition of unneeded cell growth. The result is that cells keep multiplying and form a mass of cancer tissue.

Genes are made of deoxyribonucleic acid (DNA) and, most commonly, it is damage to the DNA that results in gene malfunction to allow cancer to develop. This damage is called a mutation. Gene mutations can be inherited from parents. They can occur due to something in the environment damaging the DNA, such as carcinogens or radiation. Or a mutation can occur as a random process.

It has been estimated that 66 percent of cancer-related mutations are random; 29 percent occur due to environmental factors, such as viruses, radiation, and carcinogens; and 5 percent are inherited from parents. It requires multiple cell-control genes to be damaged before a cell will become cancerous, so not all mutations cause a cancer to develop.

Environmental factors can modify the likelihood of a random or inherited mutation causing cancer. Random mutations occur at least 10,000 times each day and are not always harmful. Beneficial mutations can occur, giving the organism a better chance of survival. This is the basis of the theory of evolution.

DNA damage occurs constantly. At the same time, the body has DNA repair processes in action. It is when these DNA repair mechanisms fail that a potentially harmful mutation in the cell can occur. With a harmful mutation, most cells simply die and are removed from the body, but some cells survive with the mutations. The ability of the body to repair damaged DNA depends on the type of cell, the age of the cell, and the tissue environment around that cell.

Repair is a complex process. For example, after DNA damage, cell cycle checkpoints are activated that pause the cell and allow time for repair to occur. Knowledge of these processes is constantly evolving.

Cancer Growth

Once a cell has undergone malignant transformation, another term for cancer development, it continues to mutate. The average breast or colon cancer has about sixty to seventy mutations that allow the cancer to grow and spread. An example is mutations that encourage the growth of blood vessels around the tumor so it can be fed nutrients from the blood.

Such mutations are occurring all the time, and those cells with new genetic changes that enhance their survival dominate. The reason why some cancers respond initially to a treatment, then become resistant, is that some cells have mutated in a way that allows them to survive the treatment.

The Immune System and Cancer

One mechanism the body uses to defend against cancer developing is by activating the immune system, a process called immune surveillance. Cancer cells contain material that the immune system recognizes as foreign, and so the immune cells, part of the body's defense system, attack these cancer cells.

The main attack comes from killer T cells in addition to natural killer cells. Unfortunately, the cancer cells are able to develop ways around this attack. For example, they can produce substances that inhibit the immune response. In recent years, there have been major advances in the development of drugs that block this cancer mechanism, allowing the immune system to better fight cancer, sometimes with dramatic success.

Cancer Metastasis

Some cancers form a mass of tumor cells in one location and do not travel elsewhere in the body, such as brain cancer (glioma). Other cancers have cells that separate from the main tumor mass and move through the body, in the lymphatic channels or through the blood. These cells can lodge in other sites, such as the lungs, liver, bones, or brain, and grow there, a process called metastasis. If the cancer cells cannot be removed by surgery or killed by radiation therapy or drug treatments, in time those cancer cells take over whole organs so the organ fails, and death results.

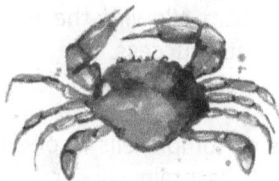

The Cancer Problem

Cancer results in an enormous amount of disease, suffering, and death worldwide. There are about seventeen million new cancer cases each year, with nearly ten million people dying from cancer annually. This means that one in every six people will die from cancer, and 70 percent of these deaths will be in low-to-middle income countries. Most deaths occur in these countries because they have larger populations and not-so-well developed cancer services.

Per head of population, however, cancer is more common in high-income Western countries. The countries with the highest rate of cancer per head of population are the Scandinavian countries, Western Europe, Australia, and South Korea. For example, the chances of someone from Mexico or Chile developing cancer is about half that of someone from Denmark or France.

Just five types of cancer account for half of all cancer cases worldwide: lung, breast, bowel, prostate, and stomach.

Cancer Type	Annual New Cases (Millions)	Percent of All Cases
Lung	2.1	12.3
Breast	2.1	12.3
Colorectal	1.8	10.6
Prostate	1.3	7.5
Stomach	1.0	6.1
Liver	0.8	5.0
Esophagus	0.6	3.4
Cervix of uterus	0.6	3.3
Thyroid	0.6	3.3
Bladder	0.5	3.2
Non-Hodgkin's lymphoma	0.5	3.0
Oral cavity	0.5	3.0
Pancreas	0.5	2.7

For men, at least one-third will get cancer at some stage in their lives—that is one in every three people, a worrying statistic. For women it is only marginally less. While the majority of cancer cases occur in older people, it can still be common in the forties and fifties. An individual's chance of getting cancer at some stage in life depends on lifestyle and where they live. Some examples are listed here.

Lung cancer in a current smoker	1 in 6
Lung cancer in a smoker quit for twenty years	1 in 30
Lung cancer in a nonsmoker	1 in 70
Breast cancer in a Western country	1 in 8
Breast cancer in China or India	1 in 16
Primary liver cancer with chronic hepatitis B	1 in 3
Primary liver cancer without hepatitis	1 in 120
Melanoma with low sun exposure (Canada)	1 in 60
Melanoma with high sun exposure (Australia)	1 in 17
Gastric cancer in Japan	1 in 13
Gastric cancer in Western countries	1 in 125

The good news is that it has been estimated that 35–40 percent of cancers can be prevented by changes you can make to your life. That is what this book is all about.

In high-income countries, the death rate for many cancers has been falling, most likely due to a combination of awareness, early detection, and improved treatments. This is little comfort. For while you might survive the cancer, you will need to go through all the treatment. Even then, you will still need to deal with ongoing anxiety about whether the cancer might recur.

The chance of a cure also depends on the type of cancer, for some are more responsive to treatment than others. Some examples of the percentage of people alive five years after diagnosis are listed here.

Testicular cancer	98 percent
Thyroid cancer	97 percent
Prostate cancer	95 percent
Breast cancer	90 percent
Hodgkin's lymphoma	86 percent
Renal and bladder cancer	75 percent

Non-Hodgkin's lymphoma	71 percent
Acute lymphocytic leukemia	68 percent
Cervical cancer	67 percent
Colorectal cancer	65 percent
Ovarian cancer	47 percent
Stomach cancer	30 percent
Esophageal cancer	19 percent
Liver and bile duct cancer	18 percent
Lung cancer	8 percent
Pancreatic cancer	8 percent
Glioblastoma (brain cancer)	4 percent

Cancer is common and can be deadly. Preventing it happening is the best option.

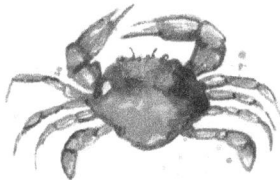

Genetics and Cancer

Cancer is a disease caused by mutation-disrupted cell-growth genes—oncogenes, tumor suppressor genes, and, to a lesser extent, DNA-repair genes. This allows uncontrolled cell multiplication and survival.

There are two types of mutations that can lead to cancer: *somatic mutations* and inherited germline mutations. The somatic mutations occur in genes that were previously structurally and functionally normal. Most somatic mutations are either spontaneous mutations or those caused by environmental factors.

Occasionally we inherit mutations from our parents, and these are called *inherited* or *germline mutations*. These mutations can result in inherited diseases, such as cystic fibrosis or muscular dystrophy. If the abnormal gene passed on from the parents is one that controls cell growth, that person will be more prone to cancer.

Having an inherited genetic mutation that makes you cancer prone does not necessarily mean you will get cancer. It takes multiple genetic mutations of the cell-control mechanisms before a cancer will develop. Inheriting one mutation gets us off to a bad start, but unless a number of somatic mutations also occur, cancer will not develop.

This accounts for why people who have inherited mutations get cancer at a younger age, as less time is needed for all the required mutations to accumulate. It also explains why not everyone with the inherited mutation will get cancer, if in their lifetime they do not accumulate enough somatic mutations to trigger a cancer.

The likelihood of cancer developing does depend on the type of inherited mutation. For example, a woman with an inherited breast cancer (BRCA) gene mutation is about twelve times more likely to develop breast cancer than someone without the mutation, but a woman with a different mutation, such as CHEK2, has only a threefold increase in risk of getting breast cancer.

That is, there are different levels of risk with different mutations. It also depends on the body organ: a woman with a BRCA1 mutation has about a 70 percent likelihood of developing breast cancer at some stage in her life, but only a 40 percent chance of developing ovarian cancer.

While we can make changes to our environment to reduce the likelihood of somatic mutations occurring, for example, reducing exposure to carcinogenic substances, we cannot do anything about any abnormal genes with which we are born. However, if you know you have an inherited mutation that makes you more prone to cancer, there are things you can do to reduce the likelihood of cancer developing. For example, you should, at a minimum, follow a lifestyle that minimizes somatic mutations. In addition, for some cancers there are medications that reduce the chances of a cancer forming. Finally, and in the extreme, it might be possible to have risk-reducing surgery to minimize cancer occurrence.

There are over fifty known inherited forms of cancer. Listed here are some of the more common cancer-forming mutations.

Inherited Breast Cancer Genes

The two major breast cancer-causing mutations are BRCA1 and BRCA2, simply standing for BReast CAncer 1 and 2. These tumor suppressor gene mutations are common and can be inherited from either parent. It has been estimated that about 1 in 400 people will have this type of mutation, and this is higher in some populations, such as Ashkenazi Jews (of Eastern European descent) where it is 1 in 40.

Women who have a BRCA1 mutation have a 70 percent chance of developing breast cancer and a 40 percent chance of developing ovarian cancer. For BRCA2, the risk is a little lower at 50 percent for breast cancer and 20 percent for ovarian cancer. The BRCA mutations account for 5–10 percent of all new breast cancers and, apart from breast and ovarian cancers, are known to be associated with an increased risk of prostate cancer, pancreatic cancer, colorectal cancer, and occasionally childhood tumors.

Testing for these genetic mutations is now relatively easy and in recent years has become less expensive. Anyone with a strong family history of breast cancer should be tested, especially if the cancer occurred at a young age or there is also a history of ovarian cancer in the family. Not surprisingly, women with a BRCA mutation often choose preventive surgery in the form of bilateral mastectomies combined with breast reconstructions. The best-known person undertaking this was actress Angelina Jolie, who had a BRCA1 mutation. While not a perfect way of preventing the disease, it does result in a major reduction in risk, as most breast tissue is removed.

There are other known inherited genetic mutations that increase breast cancer risk apart from the BRCA mutations. Medium-risk mutations include PTEN, PALB2, ATM, and CHEK2, while there are many more low-risk mutations. These low-risk mutations, called single nucleotide polymorphisms (SNP), are more common than the others but only slightly raise breast cancer risk.

A Dutch group has developed a screening test, called OncoArray, for a whole range of breast cancer susceptibility genes. This involves a blood sample that is used to screen the genome and can identify 150 or more genes that predispose to breast cancer. It includes the BRCA1 and BRCA2 mutations. It also identifies genes with a lower risk, but which are more common and so still contribute to overall breast cancer risk. This is all put together as a score, the polygenic risk score or PRS. While not in common use, it is a possibility for women who are concerned about their risk due to their family history.

The US Preventive Services Task Force recommends BRCA testing of women with a personal or family history of breast or ovarian cancers, if there are features such as breast cancer diagnosis before age fifty, bilateral breast cancer, presence of both breast and ovarian cancers, a male with breast cancer, and Ashkenazi Jewish ethnicity.

Inherited Colorectal Cancer Genes

Some people inherit a genetic mutation that makes them more susceptible to bowel cancer, accounting for about 5 percent of colorectal cancers. For the most part, these occur as part of what we call a familial syndrome, that is, where a disease pattern occurs in a family.

One of these is familial adenomatous polyposis, shortened to FAP, where family members can get large numbers of adenomatous polyps in their large bowel. Not all bowel polyps are adenomatous polyps. A pathologist needs to look through a microscope to tell what sort it is, but adenomatous polyps are an early precursor of colorectal cancer. In time, some turn malignant. This usually occurs before forty years of age.

The other main bowel cancer inherited syndrome is hereditary nonpolyposis colorectal cancer (HNPCC), also known as Lynch syndrome. In this syndrome, there is a high incidence of colorectal cancer but without the prodromal polyp formation seen in FAP. It usually appears in the forties, and these people are more prone to cancers in a number of other sites, including endometrium, ovary, stomach, kidney, brain, and skin.

The genetic mutations for these syndromes have been identified, but sometimes there are families where multiple members get colorectal cancer but a genetic mutation cannot be found. It does not mean there is no mutation, but most likely it has yet to be identified.

Li-Fraumeni Syndrome

People with this syndrome have an inherited mutation of P53, a tumor suppressor gene. It is associated with a range of cancers that start at an early age. They include breast cancer, sarcomas, brain tumors, adrenal tumors, leukemia, and lymphoma. About 50 percent of people with the P53 mutation will have developed a cancer by age thirty, and 90 percent by age seventy. Their risk is more than 100 times that of the rest of the population. Fortunately, it is rare; only about 1 in 20,000 people have it.

Finding the Cause

To prevent a disease, you need to know what causes it in the first place. You are then in a position to possibly remove that cause and so reduce the likelihood of getting the disease. Some things cannot be changed, such as inherited genetic mutations, but it has been estimated that as many as 40 percent of cancers do have a potentially modifiable cause.

Originally, it was perceptive doctors whose observations made the link between causative factors and cancer.

Galen, a Roman physician, made the observation more than 2,000 years ago that breast cancer was more common in "melancholic" women than in "sanguine" women, and postulated mood as the cause of cancer.

Sir Percival Pott, an English surgeon, linked soot on chimney sweeps as the cause of cancer of the scrotum in 1775. Most current surgeons will never have seen a case of scrotal cancer, as chimney sweeps no longer practice in the manner they did, and personal hygiene is much better.

Sir Thomas Beatson, a British surgeon, in 1896 observed that some women with advanced breast cancer, the norm at the time, went into spontaneous remission when they went through menopause. He postulated a connection between ovarian function and breast cancer. He conducted the first trial of hormone treatment for breast cancer by taking out the ovaries of a premenopausal woman with advanced breast cancer.

While demonstrating that this could be an effective treatment, the operative mortality was a terrifying 20 percent! Maybe taking this risk was still better than the inevitable early death from breast cancer? The role of hormones as a cause of breast cancer is now well-established, and hormonal treatments are an integral part of breast cancer treatment.

While the early doctors relied on observation and deduction to find causes of cancer, there is now sophisticated research methodology. In particular, determining the causes of cancers relies on epidemiological research, such as population studies, case-control studies, and long-term follow-up of large cohorts of the population.

An example of an early population study relates to breast and bowel cancers. These cancers were rare in Japan in the nineteenth century. It was assumed this was due to the inherent genes in the Japanese people protecting them from these cancers (but not stomach cancer, which was common in the Japanese). In the mid-1800s, there was migration of the Japanese to Hawaii, mainly seeking work in the cane fields. It became apparent that within a generation or two after migration, these Japanese had developed much the same rate of breast and colon cancers as the local Hawaiian population, even in those who did not intermarry.

It clearly was not genes, but changes in lifestyle after migration. There were many changes, but diet was the main difference. Hypotheses, such as the increase in meat in the diet resulted in the rise in cancer incidence, were proposed and tested by research programs.

Large prospective cohort studies provide the main evidence for the causes of cancer. In these studies, thousands of people are assessed for a range of variables. The participants complete dietary, lifestyle, and other questionnaires. Height, weight, smoking history, and blood pressure are measured. Also, they have blood samples taken and tested.

For example, the Nurses' Health Study was run by Harvard-associated institutions and involved 121,700 US nurses who were thirty to fifty-five when the study started in 1976. For the dietary component of the study, they completed food frequency questionnaires containing 130 different food items. Some blood samples were deep frozen and stored, in case new tests might be invented in the future. For example, years later telomere length, an indicator of cell health, was measured in white blood cells in the original samples. This test was not even thought about when the study was commenced.

A problem with case-control and cohort studies is bias influencing the results. People with one health-affecting behavior usually have others—a person who eats lots of fruits and vegetables is also more likely to exercise and not smoke. Separating these factors can be difficult. While statistical methods try to adjust for such behaviors, some biases can persist and so affect the results of a study.

The best research method to assess the effect of something on a disease process is a randomized controlled trial (RCT), as these sorts of studies are less likely to have inherent biases. An RCT involves recruiting a large number of people and randomly allocating half to an intervention of some sort, for example, a different diet or a weight-loss program. The other half are a control group. Both groups are followed for years to see what effect that intervention has on a disease.

This is relatively straightforward for testing a new drug, but with something like a food, it is more difficult. Can you imagine trying to convince thousands of participants that they should be randomly allocated to eating or not eating, say 100 gm of soy per day, and to continue this for at least a decade, so we can assess the health benefits of soy? Researchers have to sell the possible health benefits of soy—perhaps not all that difficult—but they have to also explain to the control half not to change their diet. If soy is possibly so good, why shouldn't they take it too? Nevertheless, such studies have been done. The Women's Health Initiative study successfully enrolled thousands of postmenopausal women and randomized half to change to a low-fat, high-fruits and vegetable diet, and continue it for many years.

The Cost of Research

Undertaking high-quality epidemiological research is labor intensive and expensive. It needs to involve large numbers of study participants, and it needs to be continued for years. Only the most motivated and best-funded researchers can do these studies, and governments might not always think this is the best way to spend their dollars.

Keep in mind, though, the possible benefits to our health as individuals and to government budgets. For example, the Women's Health Initiative study involved 160,000 participants, ran for fifteen years, and cost $625 million. The study looked at several aspects of disease and cancer causation. One of these was into the benefits and risks of using hormone replacement therapy (HRT). It has been estimated that the results from the HRT part of the study alone has since benefited the community by $37.1 billion, through lives saved, less treatment needed, and improved productivity through less time away from work.

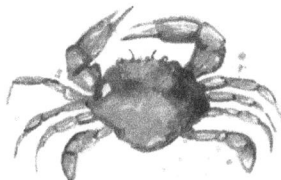

Understanding Cancer Research

Research provides the basis for our knowledge of cancer, so it is an integral part of cancer prevention and treatment. To know how to deal with the cancer problem, you must first know how the cancer functions and grows. Many millions of dollars are spent annually on cancer research. For research to be worthwhile, it must be undertaken at the highest standard: ethical, free of bias, well-planned and carried out, sufficient numbers to be meaningful, relate to human cancer, be reviewed by peers before publication, and reported honestly. Major decisions about how we manage cancer depend on this research and knowledge.

Types of cancer research include the following.

- **Molecular**—This looks at the structure and function of individual cancer cells to understand how they grow and survive. It is sometimes called basic research, although it is hardly basic, given the sophisticated techniques used.

- **Cell culture studies**—Some cancer cells, known as cell lines, can be grown in a medium that provides the nutrition they require. Drugs can be tested on these lines to give an idea if they might inhibit cancer cell growth. The original cell line used was the HeLa cancer cell line, begun in the early 1950s. HeLa was named for Henrietta Lacks, who had cervical cancer.

- **Animal experiments**—Some rats and mice develop cancers similar to humans, and these can be bred for testing of new cancer treatments. While some people object to the ethics of harming an animal, it can be argued that it is better to test drugs first on an animal, rather than a human. Potentially harmful side effects can be identified, and if the drug does not work in mice, it is not likely to work in humans.

- **Population studies**—Different populations are studied to see how their patterns of disease differ, then differences in lifestyle are sought to explain any differences.

- **Case-control studies**—Newly diagnosed cancer patients are matched with someone randomly chosen from the community. Both groups have aspects of their lifestyles, for example, diet or stress, compared by questionnaires to look for differences.

- **Longitudinal cohort studies**—These studies recruit thousands of people who have data recorded on aspects of lifestyle and diet. Blood samples are taken and stored and are followed for years to see which diseases the people in the study develop.

- **Randomized controlled trials (RCT)**—Volunteers are randomly allocated to an intervention, for example, taking a drug, implementing a weight-loss or dietary change, or being part of a control without intervention. They are then followed to see if the intervention group has a reduced occurrence of disease.

- **Meta-analyses**—Meta-analyses are studies that combine the results of a number of smaller studies, using the principle that the more people studied, the more meaningful the result. These generally include various epidemiological study types. Due to the large numbers of people included, they are a valuable means of studying cancer.

As a general rule, the further down this list of research methods, the more you can trust that any finding will be real. The pinnacle of medical research is the RCT, and the only thing that is better than an RCT is several RCTs put together in a meta-analysis. For the purposes of this book, the information here, with few exceptions, come from cohort studies, RCTs, or meta-analyses. The "in term" for such research-based information is "evidence based."

Expressing the Risk of Developing Cancer

You will find the word "risk" mentioned a lot in this book. It is easy to mix *relative* risk with *absolute* risk. An 80 percent increase in risk, the relative risk, is not an 80 percent chance of getting the disease. That is the absolute risk. For example, most people have about a one in twenty-five chance of developing colorectal cancer. Someone with a family history of colorectal cancer might have an 80 percent increase in risk. Their probability of developing it would therefore be about one in fifteen, not an 80 percent chance of getting it which would be a 1 in 1.25 chance. To keep things simple, in the book I have mostly only used the relative risk—a percentage increase or decrease in risk. Where I have used absolute risk, I have expressed it as a "one in something" chance of getting the cancer.

Don't Believe All You Read

How often do you read these words in an advertisement or on the internet? "Research shows that . . ." I cringe when I hear that, as it is often someone trying to justify some treatment, or worse, promote their own product. It might be the result from a study on ten mice, commissioned by the organization selling the product, and neither published nor peer reviewed! You can only believe "Research shows that . . ." if it has been done to an acceptably high standard, and ideally repeated by another group of researchers whose results were the same!

Part 2—The Factors

Alcohol

Cell Phones

Chronic Infections

Coffee

Diet and Cancer

Drugs to Prevent Cancer

Excess Body Fat

The Gut Microbiome

Medications to Prevent Cancer

Pesticides and Herbicides

Physical Activity

Preventive Surgery

Radiation

Smoking

Stress and Cancer

Vitamins and Minerals

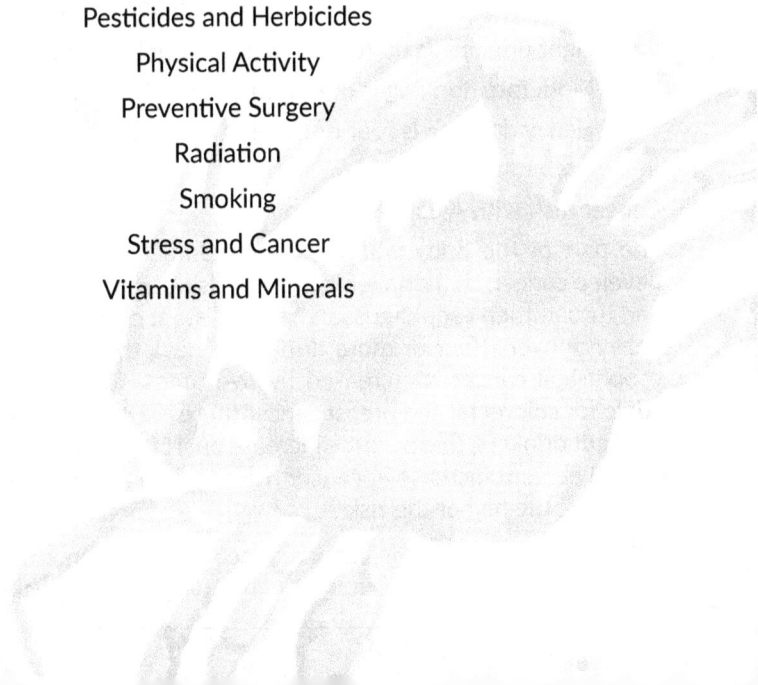

Alcohol

It has been estimated that worldwide more than 5 percent of all cancers are caused by drinking alcohol. These are mainly cancers of the gut—mouth, throat, esophagus, stomach, liver, pancreas, and bowel. In addition, alcohol consumption is recognized as a causative factor in breast cancer. The more a person drinks and the longer they have been drinking, the greater the risk of getting one of these cancers.

It doesn't seem to matter what you drink; the end result is still an increase in cancer risk, however, there are some variations. For example, in Eastern European countries, where spirits are drunk in large amounts after work, this is a factor in their high incidence of bowel cancer. In France and Italy, where wine tends to be drunk with meals, the cancer risk is lower. Nevertheless, anything more than a light alcohol intake increases the chances of getting cancer, and the popular concept that daily red wine is good for health is largely a myth.

Measuring Alcohol Consumption

A standard drink contains about 14 gm of pure alcohol. This translates into 45 ml (1.5 oz) of 40 percent proof spirits, 150 ml (5 oz) of wine that is 12 percent alcohol, and 360 ml (12 oz) of beer that is 5 percent alcohol.

- Light drinking is up to one standard drink per day.
- Moderate drinking is one to three standard drinks per day.
- Heavy drinking is four or more standard drinks per day.

Cancer Risk with Alcohol Consumption

The part of the body with the most contact with alcohol is more likely to develop cancer, so a drinker is most at risk of developing cancer of the mouth and throat, then esophagus, and more distant organs less so. For example, for heavy drinkers (four or more drinks per day), the risk for mouth, throat, and esophageal cancer is increased by five times; for liver cancer it is doubled; while for colorectal and breast cancer there is a 40–60 percent increase in risk. For light drinkers, there is little increase apart from the esophagus, where there is a 30 percent increase in cancer risk. In general, the more alcohol consumed each day, the higher the risk.

The Korean National Health Insurance Corporation has data stored on 97 percent of the Korean population, including their annual or biennial medical examinations. Data on more than 23 million adults was evaluated for alcohol consumption and the development of esophageal, gastric, and colorectal cancers over five years. There were 9,171 esophageal cancers, 135,385 gastric cancers, and 154,970 colorectal cancers. Mild-moderate drinkers were 50 percent more likely to get esophageal cancer than nondrinkers. For heavy drinkers, this was a factor of three times (300 percent increase). For heavy drinkers, there was, in addition, an increase in risk for gastric and colorectal cancer.

Esophagus. There are two different types of esophageal cancer, squamous carcinoma, and adenocarcinoma. Only squamous carcinoma is associated with alcohol consumption, and this tends to occur in the upper esophagus. Large studies have looked at the relationship between alcohol and squamous cancer of the esophagus, and virtually all confirmed that with a high intake of alcohol, the risk is significantly higher. For every 10 gm of alcohol consumed, the risk increases by 12 percent. For three standard drinks, that equates to a 50 percent increase in risk.

Stomach. Studies have shown that alcohol consumption is a significant factor in both stomach cancer development and deaths. The effect does not appear to be significant until three standard drinks or more of alcohol are consumed each day (45 gm alcohol).

Pancreas. Research into pancreatic cancer and alcohol has shown that compared to nondrinkers or light drinkers, heavy drinkers have about a 30 percent increased risk of getting pancreatic cancer, and also have a higher mortality. As with stomach cancer, this effect does not appear to start until consuming three or more drinks per day.

Colorectal. Meta-analyses have shown that alcohol increases bowel cancer risk. The risk equates to a 7 percent increase in risk per 10 gm of alcohol, so someone drinking three drinks per day (45 g) has a 30 percent increase in bowel cancer risk.

Breast. In the US Women's Health Study, 38,454 healthy women were followed for ten years, and over this time, 1,484 breast cancers developed. Drinking more than two standard drinks per day (30 gm of alcohol) was associated with a 43 percent increase in the risk of developing an invasive breast cancer, compared to nondrinkers.

How Does Alcohol Cause Cancer?

Acetaldehyde. Alcohol is not carcinogenic but it is broken down by the enzymes of the salivary glands and the liver into acetaldehyde, which is carcinogenic. This has been proven in multiple experiments. The acetaldehyde binds to DNA, damaging it, so predisposing to cancer. The acetaldehyde itself is broken down to acetate by an enzyme before it can be eliminated from the body.

Some people, especially, but not only, those of East Asian origin, have a genetically determined inactive form of this enzyme. As a consequence, acetaldehyde accumulates in these people, and they are at a particularly high risk of getting cancer from alcohol drinking. Alcohol is not just broken down to acetaldehyde in the liver; it does occur elsewhere in the body, including breast tissue and so predisposes to breast cancer.

Oxidative Stress. Alcohol can cause cancer by generating oxidized molecules that can damage DNA. Also, alcohol induced oxidative stress can result in chronic tissue inflammation.

Preventing Absorption of Antioxidants. Alcohol can prevent the absorption of cancer-preventing agents such as vitamins, folate, and carotenoids.

Estrogens. Alcohol can result in increased circulating estrogens and so increase a woman's predisposition to breast cancer.

How Much Is Too Much?

It is often said there is no safe lower level of alcohol consumption when it comes to cancer. In reality, apart from esophageal cancer, there is only minimal increase in cancer risk with light drinking, that is, on average no more than one standard alcoholic drink per day.

How much is too much depends on the cancer. For esophageal cancer, as little as one standard drink per day increases the risk, drinking one to three drinks per day increases the risk of getting breast or bowel cancer, while four or more drinks per day also results in an increased risk of getting stomach, liver, and pancreatic cancers.

There is also a direct association between the amount drunk and the risk of the cancer spreading (secondary or metastatic cancer). For cancers of the mouth and throat, for every 10 gm of alcohol drunk, the risk of spread increases by 10 percent.

What You Should Do

- Keep alcohol consumption to a minimum.

Alcohol Consumption

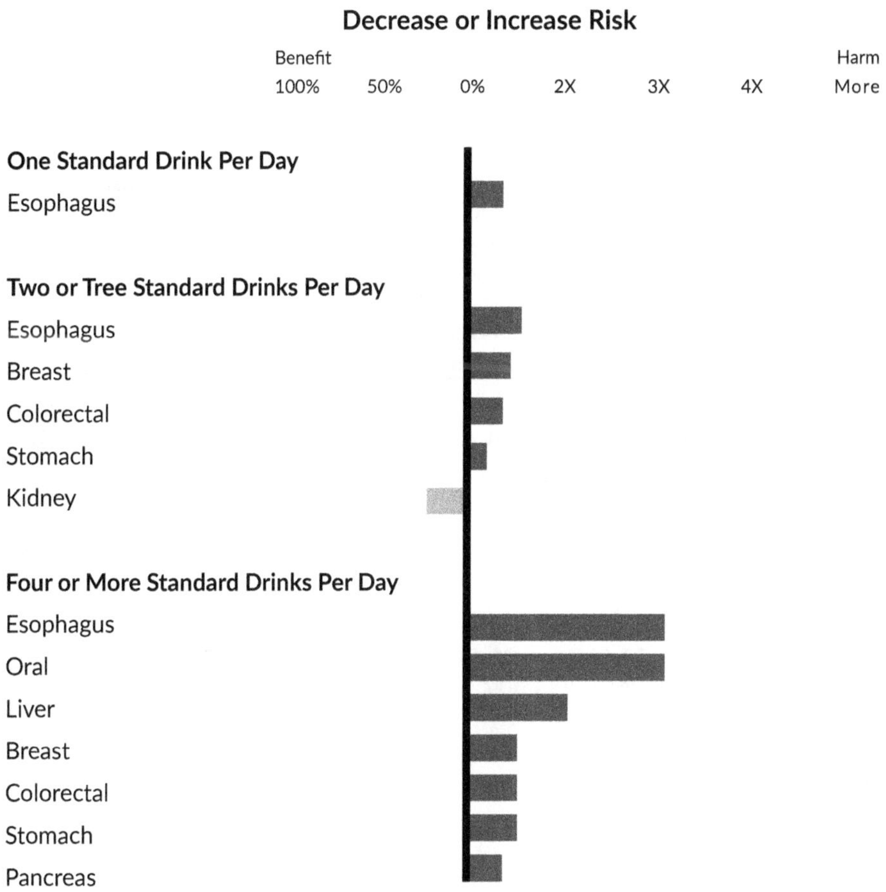

Decrease or Increase Risk

Benefit						Harm
100%	50%	0%	2X	3X	4X	More

One Standard Drink Per Day

Esophagus

Two or Tree Standard Drinks Per Day

Esophagus

Breast

Colorectal

Stomach

Kidney

Four or More Standard Drinks Per Day

Esophagus

Oral

Liver

Breast

Colorectal

Stomach

Pancreas

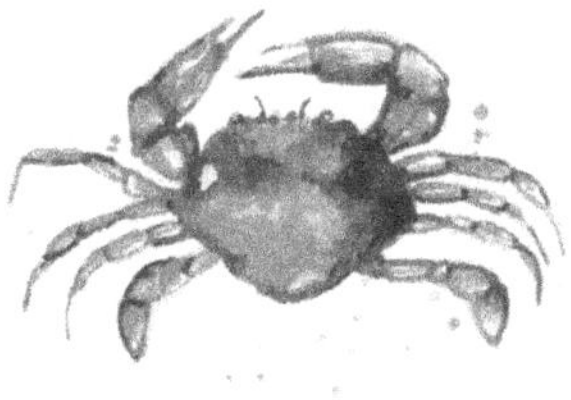

Cell Phones

The use of cell phones has expanded enormously over the past couple of decades to the point where there are now five billion cell phone users worldwide, and two-thirds of the world's population have a cell phone connection! Because cell phones are usually held to the ear and are in close proximity to the brain, there have been concerns that their use could predispose to brain tumors.

Is the Radiation from Cell Phones Harmful?

Cell phones use electromagnetic radiation in the microwave range but with a long wavelength, similar to other digital wireless systems. This type of radiation is low energy and is not sufficient to damage DNA, and there is no rational explanation as to how it could cause cancer.

The only effect of taking a call while holding the phone to your head is a miniscule temperature rise. This is less than having a cup of hot tea or coffee and is negligible. Our body temperature is constantly going through much bigger temperature swings than this.

Much of the early research was done on 2G phones that have a longer wavelength. The modern 4G and 5G phones have a shorter wavelength and so do not penetrate the head. Any energy from the waves will stay in the skin and not penetrate to the brain.

Cell Phones and Cancer

Studies in rats and mice have not shown any consistent evidence of harm from this type of radiation. In humans, if cell phones caused brain cancer, we would have seen a steady rise in the occurrence of these tumors as the use of cell phones has increased. In fact, the number of gliomas (brain cancers) has been gradually diminishing. If cell phones were a risk, we would have expected the incidence to increase by about 40 percent. The greatest risk from cell phones is texting or dialing while driving!

Since 1986, Denmark has had a centralized population register and all health data is recorded for the entire population, including cancer information. Using this information, together with that from the Danish mobile network operators, it has been possible to compare cell phone usage with cancer of the nervous system.

There were 358,403 cell phone subscribers who developed 10,729 nervous system cancers in the follow-up period from 1990 to 2007. Long-term cell phone use, ten or more years, did not increase the risk of getting brain cancer. They also looked at the duration of use, and longer use was no different than shorter use. Nor was there any change in the part of the brain the cancers were located: there was no cancer increase in that part of the brain close to the ear, near where the phone is held.

What You Should Do

- There is no need to avoid cell phone use, as there is no reason to believe it increases cancer risk.

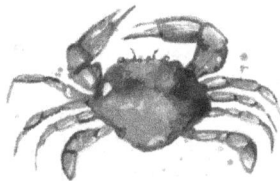

Chronic Infections

Worldwide, 17 percent of cancers occur because of a chronic infection. The main offenders are the hepatitis B and C viruses, the human papillomavirus (HPV) and the *Helicobacter pylori* organism. There are some other viruses that cause less-common cancers. Many of these infections are treatable or can be prevented by vaccination, so these cancers are mostly preventable.

Apart from causing chronic inflammation, which in itself predisposes tissues to cancer, organisms can damage cell DNA and so make the cells prone to cancerous change. Some viruses, such as HPV, make proteins that inactivate the body's tumor suppressor genes when the cell becomes infected. This is another way a virus can cause cancer.

Viruses (Oncoviruses)

Viruses that cause cancer are called oncovirses.

Human Papillomavirus. HPV is known to be an important cause of many cancers, particularly cancer of the cervix of the uterus where it is responsible for up to 90 percent of all cases. In the perineal area, it also causes cancer of the vagina, vulva, penis, anus, and rectum. In the oral cavity, it can cause cancer of the nasopharynx, tonsil, and tongue.

The virus is spread by sexual contact, by skin on skin. Rarely, it can spread from mother to baby during pregnancy. Vaccination before a person becomes sexually active is highly effective at preventing HPV-induced cancer and should be encouraged for all young men and women.

Hepatitis B. The hepatitis B virus infects the liver. With an acute infection, some people become unwell and possibly die as a result of liver failure, although others can become infected but have no illness at all.

While many people naturally eliminate the infection, some go on to develop a chronic infection that the body is unable to clear. This chronic infection of the liver can result in liver cancer, known more correctly as hepatocellular cancer.

The virus is mainly spread by blood contact, although contact from other body fluids can also spread the virus. Contact between unbroken skin, such as holding hands, does not spread the virus. The most common form of transmission of the virus is from mother to child during childbirth, particularly in countries where hepatitis B is common. Other modes of transmission include through a contaminated transfusion, reusing needles in intravenous (IV) drug users, and sexual intercourse.

Worldwide, it is estimated that about 250 million people have chronic hepatitis B infections. It is these people who are at risk of developing hepatocellular cancer. The chances of developing this liver cancer do depend on the viral load in the body, with people who have more viral activity at higher risk.

The infection is preventable by vaccination, and the World Health Organization (WHO) recommends that this course of injections starts on the first day of life in countries where it is common, and it is part of national programs in many countries. Antiviral medications can limit the extent of liver damage in chronically infected people, but the virus cannot be eradicated by medication.

Hepatitis C. The hepatitis C virus is in many ways similar to the hepatitis B virus. Both are transmitted by blood contact and both can result in an acute infection. With hepatitis B, most people clear the infection naturally with the exception of the mother-child spread disease, where most children will go on to a chronic infection.

With hepatitis C, 75–85 percent of those people infected will develop a chronic infection in the liver, and so are at risk of hepatocellular cancer. There are about 150 million people worldwide with chronic hepatitis C infection. Without treatment, up to 3 percent will develop hepatocellular cancer each year.

As opposed to hepatitis B, there is no vaccine for hepatitis C. But 95 percent of chronic infections with hepatitis C can be cured with a short course of antiviral therapy. For some cases, this is as little as eight days of medication. Such treatment of hepatitis C reduces the risk of getting hepatocellular cancer.

A French study of more than 10,000 people with chronic hepatitis C found that those who were treated were one-third less likely to get hepatocellular cancer in the following years and had a 50 percent lower chance of dying from any cause.

Anyone who is known to have a chronic hepatitis C infection should have antiviral treatment to prevent cirrhosis of the liver and to prevent liver cancer.

Other Oncogenic Viruses. Cancer caused by other viruses are much less common. They include the Epstein-Barr virus (EBV), a member of the herpes virus family, which is best known for causing glandular fever (infectious mononucleosis). It can rarely cause lymphomas, cancer of the nasopharynx, and stomach cancer. It is transmitted by saliva or genital secretions. The human T-lymphotropic virus can be associated with a rare form of lymphoma, and the Kaposi's sarcoma virus also causes a rare form of cancer. It is likely that in the future other viruses that cause cancer will be identified.

Other Chronic Infections That Cause Cancer

Chronic bacterial disease, as opposed to chronic viral disease discussed above, rarely causes cancer. The main nonviral cancer-causing organism is *Helicobacter pylori*. It can result in stomach infection and cancer.

Helicobacter pylori. Many people have *Helicobacter pylori* in their gut. However, most people with this infection have no symptoms so do not know that they have it. In some people, the organism causes a chronic infection called chronic gastritis. This can result in nausea and pain. Taking a biopsy of the stomach lining and testing it for *Helicobacter pylori* is normal practice, if an endoscopy of the stomach is done to investigate nausea or pain. In addition to causing stomach cancer, there is some evidence that *Helicobacter pylori* can increase the chances of getting colorectal cancer, also a form of lymphoma of the stomach lining.

Elimination of *Helicobacter pylori* from the stomach by a course of antibiotics reduces the chances of getting stomach cancer. A randomized trial of 2,258 people in China with *Helicobacter pylori* infection found that those randomized to a two-week course of treatment subsequently developed stomach cancer at only half the rate of those who were not treated, with the benefit persisting for more than twenty years. Vaccines against *Helicobacter pylori* are being developed but are not yet available. These are needed, as the organism is developing resistance to the commonly used antibiotics. The organisms in yogurt tend to suppress the *Helicobacter pylori* and eating yogurt might help in treatment.

Should everyone be tested for *Helicobacter pylori* infection, and if infected, then treated? The tests are simple and are either a breath test or a stool test. In Western populations, such testing is not generally recommended as the risk of developing stomach cancer is low, only 1–2 percent over a lifetime. Stomach cancer risk is considerably higher in Asian populations, and some Japanese authorities do *Helicobacter pylori* screening of all high school students, treating those with a proven infection.

There is some evidence that this organism does have some beneficial effects in reducing allergies, reflux, and inflammatory bowel disease.

What You Should Do

- Encourage all adolescents to be vaccinated for HPV before they become sexually active.
- Vaccinate children at birth for hepatitis B, when the mother is a carrier of the virus.
- Vaccinate people at high risk for hepatitis B, such as IV drug users and healthcare workers.
- Someone who is known to have the hepatitis C virus should have it treated by oral antiviral drugs, with a good chance of cure.
- Anyone with a known *Helicobacter pylori* infection should have the infection treated.

Treating Chronic Infections

Decrease or Increase Risk

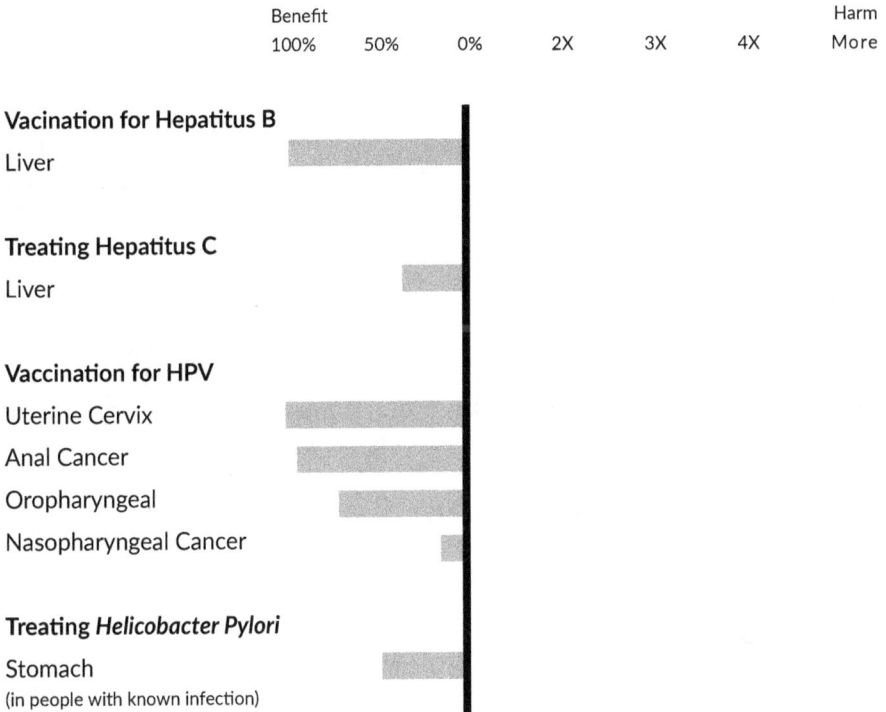

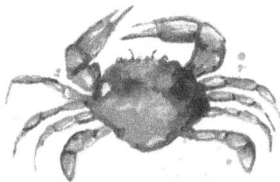

Benefit						Harm
100%	50%	0%	2X	3X	4X	More

Vacination for Hepatitus B

Liver

Treating Hepatitus C

Liver

Vaccination for HPV

Uterine Cervix

Anal Cancer

Oropharyngeal

Nasopharyngeal Cancer

Treating *Helicobacter Pylori*

Stomach
(in people with known infection)

Coffee

There is a sad rule about food that says that if it tastes good, then it is bad for you. Well, when it comes to coffee, the converse is true. As most people drink coffee, that's great news. There is evidence that coffee drinkers, especially those in the three to four cups per day bracket, have a reduced chance of dying from a whole range of diseases.

Coffee and Survival

In one US study, over 90,000 adults without cancer or cardiovascular disease at baseline were surveyed from 1998 to 2001, and followed for twelve years. Over this time, about 10 percent of the study population died. After adjusting for smoking and other possible confounding factors, those who drank three or more cups of coffee each day had a 20 percent reduction in their chances of dying from any cause compared to non- or low-coffee drinkers, and this applied to decaffeinated and caffeinated coffee. This was mainly by preventing heart disease, respiratory disease, and diabetic deaths.

Since the US study, there has been a larger European study covering ten countries. The European Prospective Investigation into Cancer and Nutrition (EPIC) had a longer follow-up of the study population. The findings were overall similar in that people with a high coffee intake had about a 10 percent reduction in death, mainly from gastrointestinal disease and respiratory diseases. Coffee was particularly protective for death from liver disease.

Coffee and Cancer

Biliary Cancers

The best evidence is for cancer of the gallbladder and biliary tracts (the ducts that lead out of the liver and gallbladder). A Swedish study of 72,680 men and women found that, compared to those who drank one or less cups of coffee per day, those drinking three cups halved their chances of developing this sort of cancer, while those drinking four or more cups per day had a 60 percent reduction. The cause of gallbladder and bile duct cancer is not well understood, but having gallstones increases this risk. Coffee stimulates the gallbladder to empty bile, and this results in less exposure of the gallbladder to the bile, also less gallstone formation.

Liver Cancer

Coffee also reduces the risk of primary liver cancer (hepatocellular cancer). In Western countries, this cancer is relatively uncommon, but in Eastern Asian countries it is one of the commonest cancers due to chronic hepatitis infections. In the EPIC study, liver cancer deaths were almost halved in those who had a high coffee intake.

Colon Cancer

A case-control study from Israel of nearly 10,000 people found that coffee consumption was associated with a 26 percent reduction in colorectal cancer risk. The highest group of coffee drinkers, more than 2.5 cups per day, had the greatest benefit, and it applied to both caffeinated and decaffeinated coffee.

Prostate Cancer

Coffee drinking is associated with a reduced risk of prostate cancer. The Health Professionals Follow-up Study in the US followed almost 50,000 men who regularly reported on their coffee consumption. Some 5,000 cases of prostate cancer developed in these men during follow-up.

Men who consumed six or more cups per day had a 20 percent reduction in their chances of getting any sort of prostate cancer and a 60 percent reduction in lethal prostate cancer. Drinking one to three cups per day was associated with a 30 percent reduction in lethal prostate cancer. These benefits applied to both caffeinated and decaffeinated coffee.

Cancer of the Endometrium of the Uterus

Coffee also reduces endometrial cancer. The Swedish Mammography Cohort study followed 60,000 women for nearly eighteen years, and during this time 677 women developed endometrial cancer. Being overweight or obese are known risk factors for endometrial cancer. For these women, drinking four or more cups of coffee per day reduced their endometrial cancer risk by 25 percent.

How Does Coffee Prevent Cancer?

Bioactive Compounds in Coffee

Coffee contains a lot of biologically active compounds, including polyphenols, diterpenes, and caffeine. Some of these have been linked to lower levels of inflammation and insulin resistance, while some are antimutagenic or antioxidant. The level of these active compounds varies with the type of coffee bean, the amount of roasting, brewing techniques, and serving size.

Improved Insulin Sensitivity

Coffee consumption improves insulin sensitivity. Both caffeinated and decaffeinated coffee are associated with reduced insulin levels, particularly among overweight women. Insulin and insulin sensitivity are factors in cancer development.

Improved Liver Function

Measurement of liver enzymes indicates that coffee drinkers have lower enzyme levels than nondrinkers, indicating improved liver function. Experimental studies show that coffee acts on liver cells by lowering proliferation and stimulating apoptosis, both being anticancer actions.

Fewer Gallstones

Coffee stimulates the gallbladder to contract and empty bile, so there is less stasis and gallstone formation. Gallstones are known to be associated with gallbladder cancer.

How Much Is Enough?

Coffee drinking, especially in the three cups per day or more range, significantly reduces a person's chances of getting a range of cancers. Drinking more is better. Some studies have shown that this applies to both caffeinated and decaffeinated coffee, while in other studies, it was just caffeinated coffee that produced the benefit. It also has other health benefits as manifested by a reduced death rate from respiratory, heart, and gastrointestinal diseases, and diabetes.

What You Should Do

- For coffee lovers the answer is easy: just drink at least three cups per day.
- If you find coffee keeps you awake, there is evidence decaffeinated coffee is also beneficial, or drink your coffee before midday.
- If you do not drink coffee, the health benefits would make it worth trying to change.

Drinking Coffee (Three or More Cups Per Day)

Decrease or Increase Risk

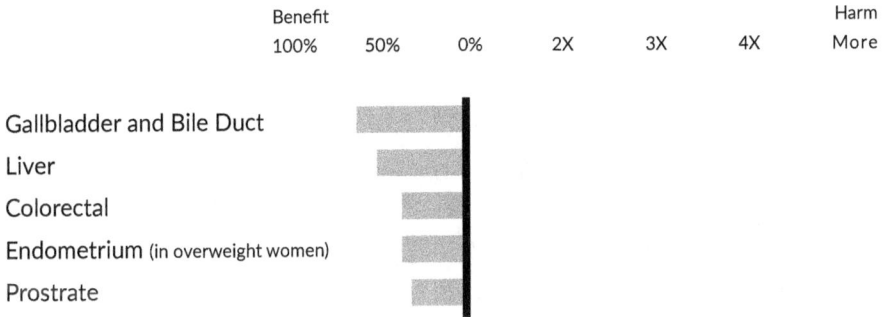

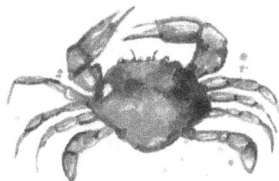

	Benefit						Harm
	100%	50%	0%	2X	3X	4X	More

Gallbladder and Bile Duct

Liver

Colorectal

Endometrium (in overweight women)

Prostrate

Diet and Cancer

Food contains many bioactive substances, some potentially beneficial and some toxic and possibly carcinogenic. It would surprise no one that what we eat could have a significant influence on whether we develop cancer at some stage in our lives. It has been estimated that about 30 percent of cancers can be prevented by eating a healthy diet. Because of the complexity of diets and foods, it has been difficult for research to find which foods cause, or prevent, cancer. There are still many unknowns.

What Is Food?

You might think, "What a silly question—food is what we put in our mouths to keep us going." That is true, but what we put in our mouths does not stay that way for long. The body has an effective digestive process to break down undigested food. For example, if we eat an orange, before long, it is no longer an orange. It is sugars, fiber, vitamins, and minerals, and what the body does with it depends on a lot of factors.

If we are exercising, the sugars might be put straight into the bloodstream for the muscles to turn into energy. But if not, then the sugars are sent to the liver for storage for when we might need energy later. The vitamin C could be utilized for cell function, but if we have had our fill of vitamin C already, it might be sent straight to the kidney for excretion.

If body function is not optimum, say the person has celiac disease or low gastric acidity, both common situations, then the digestive process might not be so effective. So, if you are considering diet and how it might influence the body, it is not simply a matter of what you put in, is what you get.

Foods are also highly complex. A handful of beans is not just some protein, sugars, vitamins, and fiber. It comprises hundreds of different compounds, many of which have some biological activity in our body and so have the possibility of changing the way our body functions. Understanding their structure, and working out how they interact with our bodies, is poorly understood.

Furthermore, it is likely that it takes years of eating a particular food for it to influence cancer development. Having a binge last week of fruits and vegetables will not stop you getting cancer. You have to keep it up for years to provide even a small benefit. Thus, for any research into the association between diet and cancer to truly reflect the effect of a food, it needs to run for many years.

Measuring Diet

Measuring what we eat is difficult and often inaccurate. There are two main techniques, the *food frequency questionnaire* (FFQ) and the *dietary diary* or *record*. The FFQ asks you to recall from a long list of foods how often you eat, and how much you would normally eat, on each occasion. For example, how often you eat potatoes and how big a serving you normally eat. This is not easy, especially when there are pages of questions, and people have notoriously poor recollections of what they would normally eat.

The other method, the dietary record, is more accurate but still has problems. For example, everything you eat for a week or two is recorded, either in a diary or by photograph. You are also asked to give an idea of the weight or volume. These data need to be entered into a computer to be converted to individual foods, food groups, and even individual nutrients. Apart from the inaccuracy of remembering what you have eaten during the day, when you finally get time to fill in the diary, it also relies on honesty and there might be a guilt factor. We just might forgo the ice cream we normally have after the market on Saturdays, as it wouldn't look good in the dietary diary!

Another reason the study of food is not easy is that anything we eat will affect what else we might eat. For example, if we put some extra olive oil into our cooking, that seems simple enough, but oils contain a lot of energy and almost certainly you will not feel the need to eat so much other food. You might not have room for that snack you were thinking about at the end of a meal. It is easier, and more sensible in many ways, to study a diet or a dietary pattern, rather than a single food.

The Major Dietary Studies

Most of the quality information we have about diet and cancer comes from either *dietary intervention studies* or *prospective cohort studies*. In a dietary intervention study, healthy individuals are recruited, then randomized, so that one group makes a specific change in their diet; this change being something that we would hope would result in less future disease. The other group continues their normal diet and so are the controls.

The groups are monitored over time for adherence to the dietary change and disease development, as it is often years later that any benefit is apparent. Once demonstrated beyond doubt, the whole population can be advised to make this change in their diet. This is the best form of dietary study, but doing such studies is difficult, and so there have only ever been a few large-scale dietary intervention studies.

A prospective cohort study of diet and cancer asks a large number of people in good health to have data about themselves recorded, including food consumption. They are followed for years to see what diseases they might develop. Researchers can then look back on the original information and see what was different between the group who developed a particular disease, and those who did not. From this, they get an idea of what might have caused the disease.

Some of the main dietary studies are listed here.

The **Women's Health Initiative** (WHI) study contained both dietary intervention and cohort study components. It looked at how dietary change might affect disease development in postmenopausal women. Starting in 1991, it enrolled more than 160,000 women, ages fifty to seventy-nine, over a period of fifteen years. Until then, research into disease had largely focused on white males and this was part of a push to involve women. The dietary modification part of the study aimed to see if change to a low-fat diet would help reduce the development of breast and colorectal cancers, also heart disease, stroke, and osteoporosis.

The **Linxian Nutrition Intervention Trial**. Linxian in China has one of the highest rates of cancer of the esophagus and stomach in the world. In the trial, thousands of people at high risk of developing these cancers were randomized to take combinations of vitamins and minerals or a placebo. After five years, the rates of cancer in the groups were compared.

The **Women's Healthy Eating and Living** (WHEL) **Study** and the **Women's Intervention Nutritional Study** (WINS) randomized women who had been diagnosed with breast cancer to a specified dietary change or not. In the WINS, it was to reduce fat to 15 percent of energy intake, while the WHEL study encouraged a healthy eating pattern of fruits, vegetables, and fiber with fat reduced to 20 percent. The studies looked at recurrence and survival.

The **Nurses' Health Study** is a prospective cohort study. It enrolled 121,700 US nurses who were thirty to fifty-five when the study started in 1976. For the dietary component of the study, they completed food frequency questionnaires containing 130 different food items. It has been one of the most important sources of information about the cause of disease of all time, with hundreds of research papers resulting from analysis of the information gained.

The **Health Professionals Follow-Up Study**. This study was designed to complement the Nurses' Health Study but with the focus of male health, recruiting over 50,000 male health professionals.

The **European Prospective Investigation into Cancer and Nutrition** (EPIC) study enrolled more than 500,000 participants from ten European countries, starting in 1992. Detailed questionnaires were completed, measurements taken, and blood samples collected and stored.

The **NutriNet-Santé** study is a French-based cohort study where participants are recruited over the internet, filling in their data online. They are followed by internet questionnaires to record any diseases they might develop over the following years.

Foods That Could Prevent or Cause Cancer

Fruits and Vegetables

Fruits and vegetables contain a whole variety of chemical compounds, called phytochemicals, which are potentially cancer-preventing. These include the majority of the vitamins. Many of these phytochemicals can scavenge and remove the free oxygen radicals that can cause cancer, these substances are known as antioxidants. Also, there are flavonoids that can inhibit cancer-forming enzymes, isoflavones that can reduce estrogen stimulation of tissues, indoles, allium compounds, phenols, and many more. In addition to these phytochemicals, fruits and vegetables are a good source of fiber, and this might also have a protective effect.

Protection from cancer by a diet rich in fruits and vegetables has been shown in many studies, and the results have been pooled to allow a more robust analysis. This pooled analysis, which resulted in more than 750,000 people being included, concluded that people who eat 800 gm or more of fruits and vegetables per day had a 25 percent lower risk of getting cancer of the lower colon than those eating less than 200 gm per day. A similar type of study, looking at breast cancer, found that women who ate a lot of fruits and vegetables had a nearly 20 percent lower risk than those who did not eat many fruits and vegetables.

Fat

It was once thought that eating saturated fats could increase the risk of getting cancer. This suggestion came from the observation that countries where a high-fat diet was common had a higher rate of certain cancers than countries where a low-fat consumption was the norm. For example, bowel and breast cancers were uncommon in Japan early in the nineteenth century, but common in the US. When Japanese migrated to the US, their rate of getting these cancers gradually increased as they changed to a Western lifestyle. One of these changes was an increase in the amount of saturated fat in the diet, hence the saturated fat cancer hypothesis. Large cohort studies, and one large intervention study, have for the most part disproven any relationship.

In the dietary modification component of the Women's Health Initiative study, nearly 50,000 women were randomized to either reduce the amount of fat in their diet or continue with their usual diet. The aim was to reduce fat intake to 20 percent of total caloric intake. For the most part, this group successfully maintained the dietary change for the duration of the study. There was no significant reduction in the rate of colon or breast cancer development after eight years of dietary fat reduction.

The outcomes of the women who took part in this study were reviewed recently, with sixteen years having elapsed, so there is a much longer follow-up, and in particular looking at deaths from breast cancer. Of the original

50,000 participants, deaths overall were less in the dietary modification group (234 compared to 443). This was a combination of a reduction in breast cancer deaths and fewer deaths from heart disease. Furthermore, the breast cancers that did develop in the reduced-fat diet women were less aggressive.

Overall, pooled cohort studies have not shown any good link between dietary fat and any cancer, so apart from the data relating to breast cancer mortality above, dietary fat is no longer considered a risk factor for cancer.

Meat

Meat consists largely of protein and fat, and these are not considered to be carcinogenic. When cooked at high temperatures, however, meat can form chemicals, such as amines and polycyclic hydrocarbons, that have been shown to be cancer-forming in animal studies. Processed meats are more of a concern, as they usually contain nitrates and nitrites that are used in the preserving process. In the stomach the nitrates and nitrates are converted into carcinogenic N-nitroso compounds.

For red meat, it has been estimated that the risk of colorectal cancer increases by 17 percent for every 100 gm eaten on average each day. For processed meats, such as ham and salamis, the risk of getting colorectal, pancreatic, or prostate cancer increases by 20 percent for every 50 gm consumed on average per day. Eating a 200 gm steak or equivalent of red meat per day would therefore increase the likelihood of developing colorectal cancer from one in twenty-four (in a Western population), to about one in eighteen.

Fiber

Eating a diet rich in fiber is thought to be protective against cancer development, with benefit through a number of mechanisms. For a start, dietary fiber is fermented by the bacteria in the bowel to short-chain fatty acids, and these are antiproliferative. Fiber also increases stool bulk, which means it transits through the colon more rapidly, and so any carcinogens in the stool have less contact time with the bowel wall. High-fiber diets also reduce insulin resistance, something that has been linked to a number of cancers.

The EPIC study of more than 500,000 people done in a number of European countries found that, compared to people who did not eat much fiber, those who ate the most almost halved their risk of getting colorectal cancer. A meta-analysis of other cohort studies estimated that for every 10 gm of fiber eaten on average each day, the risk of colorectal cancer decreases by 10 percent. The problem with studying fiber intake, however, is that it is difficult to separate the effect of the fiber from that of its sources, cereals, fruit, and vegetables. Is it the fiber, or is it the fruits, vegetables, or grains that provide the protection?

Whole Grains

The outer part of whole grains, the bran and the germ, are the main sources of protein, fiber, vitamins, and minerals, such as selenium, zinc, and copper.

Unfortunately, most of this valuable part of cereal is lost in processing, the remainder being mostly carbohydrate. In addition, these outer cereal layers contain phytoestrogen lignans and phenolic compounds that have potentially anticancer actions. The outer whole grain also helps slow digestion and so there is less rise in insulin.

The benefit of whole-grain consumption is best seen in colorectal cancer, where combined analyses of multiple studies have shown a 10–20 percent decrease in colorectal cancer for people with a high intake of whole grains.

Fish and Marine Fatty Acids

Traditional Inuit populations who lived on a marine-based diet had a low incidence of breast and prostate cancers. As their diets became more Westernized, the rates of these cancers have increased, leading to the idea that the marine oils they ate could have been protective. Marine-derived fatty acids, also known as omega-3 fatty acids—primarily eicosapentaenoic acid and docosahexaenoic acid, have been shown to reduce inflammation and so might reduce cancer.

Studies have shown that people who eat fish have a lower chance of getting colorectal cancer, with about a 10 percent reduction if they eat on average 100 gm of fish per day. Unfortunately, trials of marine-oil supplements have not shown any benefit. A meta-analysis was carried out on nineteen trials that had compared omega-3 supplementation with a placebo and involving 68,954 people. There was a total of 1,039 cancer events, but no reduction in cancer incidence in those taking the fish oil. In fact, there was a small, but not statistically significant, increase in cancer. In the vitamin D and omega-3 trial (VITAL), 25,871 people were randomized to take either fish oil or a placebo for five years. Of these, 1,617 developed cancer with 342 cancer deaths. Again, there was no reduction either in the incidence of cancer or in deaths from cancer among those who took the fish oil.

Dairy Products

Dairy products are an important source of calcium, lactic acid producing bacteria in fermented milk products such as yogurt, and other bioactive chemicals such as butyrates. Calcium is essential for cell function, including regulating cell growth and differentiation, and so has the potential to influence cancer development. Lactic acid producing bacteria influence the biome, the vast numbers of gut bacteria and so possibly colorectal cancer, while butyrate also has a potential colorectal cancer prevention role.

Studies have shown that people who eat dairy products have a lower risk of developing colorectal cancer. The risk progressively diminishes for every 100 gm consumed each day, until at 500 gm per day, the risk is reduced by 20 percent compared to someone who has little dairy consumption.

There is also consistent evidence from studies of dairy intake and breast cancer that there is benefit from higher consumption of dairy. For prostate cancer, however, the opposite applies with men who consume a diet rich in dairy having a 10 percent increase in prostate cancer risk compared to low consumers.

Phytoestrogens

Phytoestrogens first came to prominence in the 1940s, when sheep were found to become infertile for no apparent reason. Research tracked the problem to new clovers that had been introduced to farming to improve the quality of pasture for livestock. The clovers were rich in phytoestrogens and these resulted in multicystic ovaries in the sheep fed on these pastures.

As the name indicates, phyto means plant, these are naturally occurring estrogens that are found in some plants, particularly soy, clover, and the outer part of cereals but also in fruits and vegetables. There are a number of different types, with the main types being isoflavones, from soy and clover, and lignans, that are found in the outer coating of cereals. While these are weak estrogens, perhaps only a thousandth the strength of oestradiol, the body's own estrogen, they are absorbed in vast numbers once eaten.

The theory is that while weak, their sheer numbers are enough to occupy some of the estrogen receptors on breast cells and other cells and so prevent the body's own estrogen entering. That way, they might act like a natural antiestrogen and so prevent breast or other hormone-influenced cancers, such as uterus and ovary. They are also antioxidants and inhibit the enzyme CYP1A1, which results in decreased carcinogen metabolites.

Soy is the most important source of isoflavones. Asian populations consume much more soy than Western people. This high soy intake in Asian women has been shown to be associated with a reduced breast cancer risk. Another way of assessing phytoestrogen consumption is to look at excretion in the urine, as this mirrors the amount eaten. In case-control studies, Chinese women with breast cancer have been shown to have lower amounts of both isoflavones and lignans in their urine compared to matched controls. A study in Western women found similar results but measured blood levels instead of urine.

Phytoestrogens have been shown to be protective for lung cancer, although this only applies to people who have never smoked. Those with the highest consumption of phytoestrogens had a 34 percent reduction in their risk of getting lung cancer compared to those with the lowest consumption.

There is also evidence to suggest that phytoestrogen consumption might reduce the risk of both endometrial and ovarian cancers.

Sugars and Glycemic Load

Some carbohydrates are absorbed rapidly and quickly raise the blood sugar levels. This results in an insulin spike. Such foods are called high glycemic foods or high glycemic index (GI) foods. Examples of high GI foods are added sucrose or fructose in drinks or foods, white bread, white rice, potatoes, cakes, and many packaged breakfast cereals. Not all carbohydrates behave like this.

Whole grains, beans, low-fat dairy, nuts, and most fruits and vegetables are digested slowly and so are low GI foods. Long-term eating of high GI foods results in high insulin levels, a situation called insulin resistance, as the tissues no longer respond to insulin in the normal manner. Sugar in the blood no longer enters the cells as it did, and blood sugar rises. This situation can lead to diabetes. It also increases the availability of insulin-like growth factor 1 (IGF-1), a promoter of cell growth and division. This increases the possibility of genetic mutations occurring, leading to cancer.

High levels of IGF-1 have been shown to be associated with an increased risk of colorectal, breast, endometrial, pancreatic, and prostate cancers. Large cohort studies have shown that both men and women who have the highest levels of IGF-1 in their blood have an increase in their risk of getting colorectal cancer. Similarly, in relation to people with the highest IGF-1 levels, men have a more than fourfold increase in prostate cancer risk, and women have a more than doubling of their breast cancer risk, especially younger women.

A high glycemic load is also associated with an increased risk of cancer of the endometrium. The Women's Health Initiative cohort study measured insulin resistance in more than 22,000 postmenopausal women and followed them for eighteen years. Death from any cancer was 25 percent higher in the women with the highest levels of insulin resistance.

Fructose in the form of corn syrup is commonly added as a sweetener to processed foods. Fructose consumption and pancreatic cancer are linked and, for every 25 gm of fructose consumed on average each day, the risk of developing pancreatic cancer rises by more than 20 percent. A can of soda drink contains about 37 gm of fructose, so could increase pancreatic cancer risk by 30 percent, from one in sixty-five (in a Western population) to about one in fifty.

Dietary Patterns and Cancer

Traditional Mediterranean Diet

The traditional Mediterranean diet is characterized by a high intake of seafood, vegetables, fruits, nuts, and legumes. There is also a high intake of olive oil and a low intake of saturated fats. There is little consumption of dairy products, meat, and poultry, but there is a regular but moderate intake of wine, mainly with meals. This sort of diet is common in countries bordering the Mediterranean Sea and so has been called the Mediterranean diet. It is recognized as being associated with better health and longevity.

There have been a number of trials where outcomes after change to a Mediterranean diet have been examined. These have primarily looked at heart disease, but the subsequent development of cancer has also been studied. In one such study from Spain, over 4,000 women were randomized to change to either a Mediterranean diet supplemented by taking extra olive oil, a Mediterranean diet supplemented by nuts, or a control diet. After five years, the Mediterranean diet subjects had developed fewer breast cancers compared to the control diet subjects who had just been asked to reduce the amount of fat in their diet.

A meta-analysis of eighty-three studies of a Mediterranean diet and cancer has been done, which included more than two million study subjects, mostly from cohort studies. This showed that people who ate a diet close to a Mediterranean diet had a lower chance of developing cancer. This group had a 15 percent lower chance of getting colorectal cancer, about a 10 percent lower chance of getting breast cancer, and overall there was a 14 percent lower chance of dying from any sort of cancer.

Ultra-Processed Diets

Ultra-processed foods tend to have poorer nutritional quality, containing more salt, sugar, fat, less fiber, and fewer micronutrients. In addition, they are associated with a higher glycemic response.

The NutriNet-Santé prospective cohort study recruited more than 100,000 healthy volunteers from the internet and investigated possible associations between the consumption of ultra-processed foods and cancer. The amount of ultra-processed food in the diet was calculated from dietary records, and the main contributors were sugary foods (26 percent) and sugary drinks (20 percent), ultra-processed starchy foods and cereals (16 percent), and ultra-processed fruits and vegetables (15 percent).

Within five years, 2,228 people had developed cancer. Overall, those with the highest consumption of ultra-processed foods had a 20 percent increased risk of getting any cancer. The main affect was a 50 percent increase in colorectal cancer, and a 30 percent increase in postmenopausal breast cancer.

Vegetarian Diets

Vegetarians have long been thought to get less cancer than meat eaters. This has been confirmed in a study of 61,566 men and women recruited in the 1980s and 1990s in the UK, who were followed for twelve years. There were 32,403 meat eaters, 8,562 nonmeat eaters who did eat fish, and 20,601 vegetarians. During the follow-up period, 3,350 developed some form of cancer.

The vegetarians and fish eaters had a lower rate of developing most cancers, but in particular they had about a 70 percent reduction in stomach cancer, a 40–60 percent reduction in ovarian cancer, a 20–50 percent reduction in bladder cancer, and a 15–45 percent reduction in lymphomas and leukemias. Overall, fish eaters had an 18 percent reduction in cancer, and vegetarians had a 12 percent cancer reduction.

Proinflammatory or "Western" Diet

There is no strict definition of what constitutes a "Western" diet, but in general it includes red and processed meats, refined grains, and sugary drinks. It is often referred to as a proinflammatory diet, because it can result in low-grade and long-term inflammation in the body, a known mechanism for cancer development.

One study followed 121,050 adults over twenty-six years. They had their diet assessed at the start and every four years during the study period. It found that men who ate a proinflammatory diet were 40 percent more likely to develop colorectal cancer, and for women the risk was a 20 percent increase.

What You Should Do

You can reduce your chances of developing and dying from cancer by ensuring that most of what you eat consists of these foods.

- Fruits and vegetables
- Whole grains
- Fiber
- Dairy
- Fish

Minimize your consumption of these foods.

- Meats, especially processed meats
- High glycemic foods, such as sugary foods and highly processed cereals

Diet—Foods

Decrease or Increase Risk

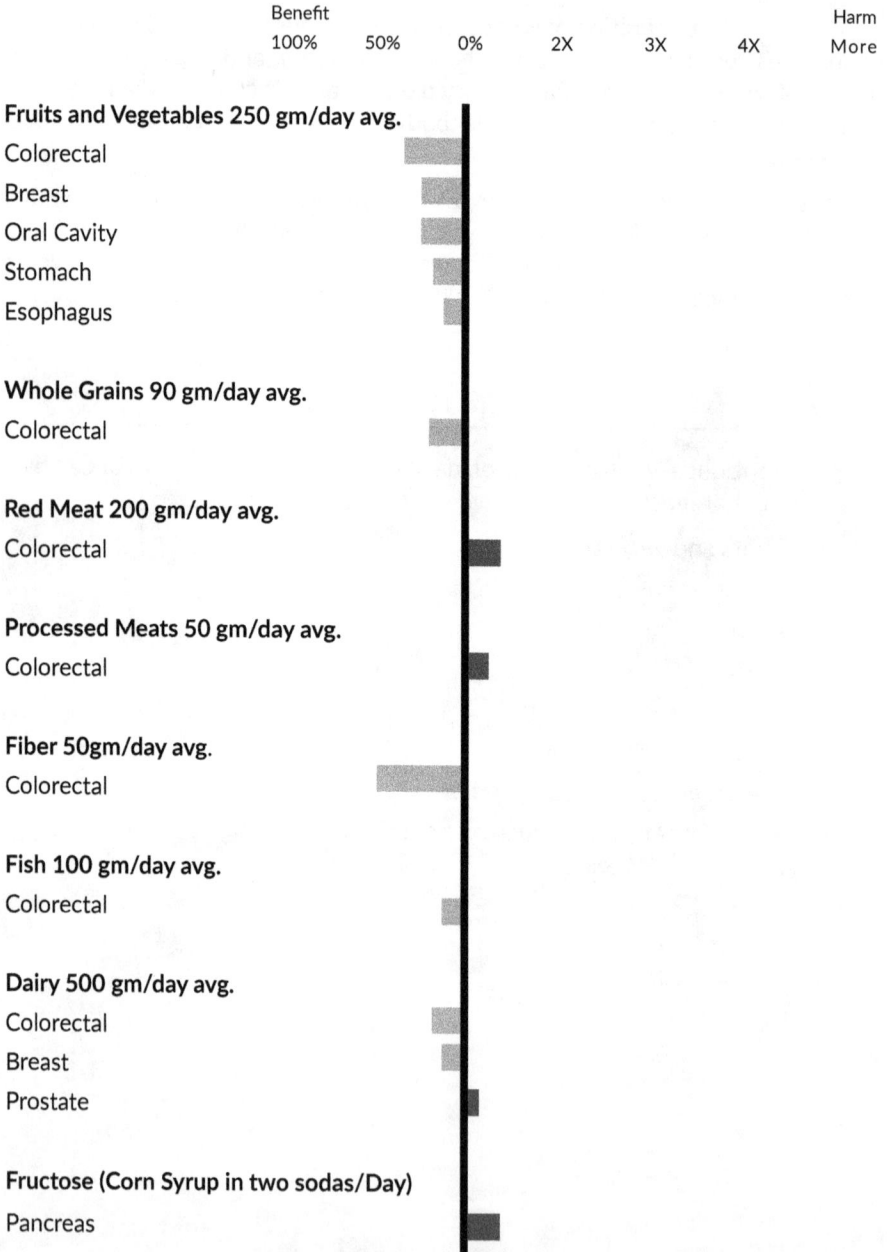

Benefit						Harm
100%	50%	0%	2X	3X	4X	More

Fruits and Vegetables 250 gm/day avg.
Colorectal
Breast
Oral Cavity
Stomach
Esophagus

Whole Grains 90 gm/day avg.
Colorectal

Red Meat 200 gm/day avg.
Colorectal

Processed Meats 50 gm/day avg.
Colorectal

Fiber 50gm/day avg.
Colorectal

Fish 100 gm/day avg.
Colorectal

Dairy 500 gm/day avg.
Colorectal
Breast
Prostate

Fructose (Corn Syrup in two sodas/Day)
Pancreas

Diet—Dietary Patterns

Decrease or Increase Risk

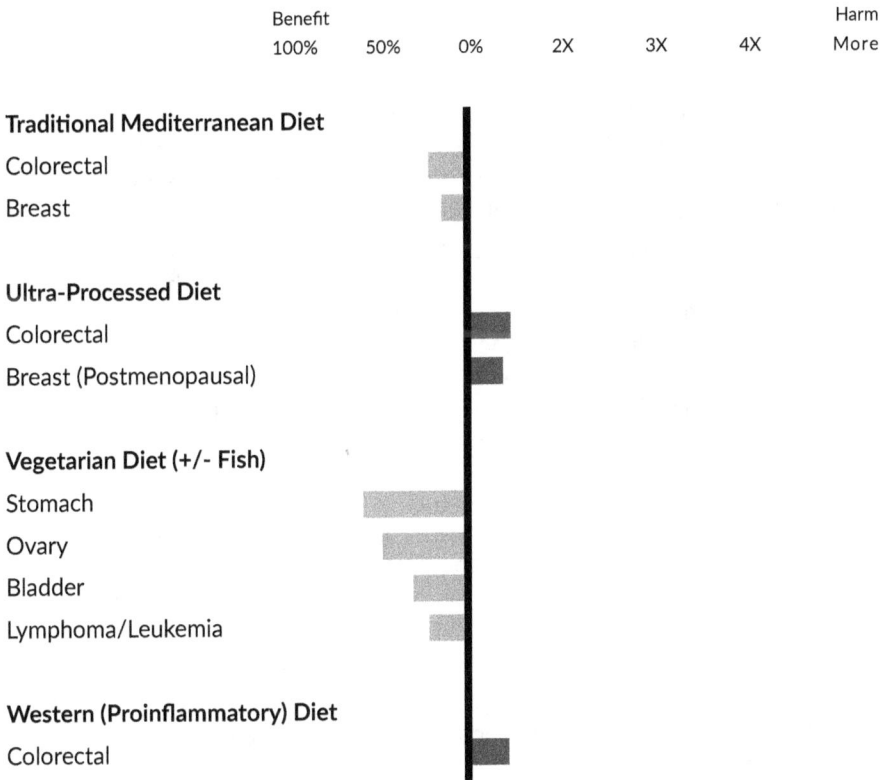

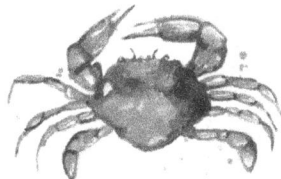

Benefit						Harm
100%	50%	0%	2X	3X	4X	More

Traditional Mediterranean Diet

Colorectal

Breast

Ultra-Processed Diet

Colorectal

Breast (Postmenopausal)

Vegetarian Diet (+/- Fish)

Stomach

Ovary

Bladder

Lymphoma/Leukemia

Western (Proinflammatory) Diet

Colorectal

Excess Body Fat

Having excess body fat is not good for health. It increases the chances of getting a whole range of diseases, the most common and lethal of which is ischemic heart disease. There is no doubt that it significantly increases the chances of getting, and dying from, cancer.

The International Agency for Research on Cancer (IARC), in a review of the preventive effects of weight control on cancer risk, found that obesity can cause at least 14 cancers—esophageal adenocarcinoma, gastric cardia, colon and rectum, liver, gallbladder, pancreas, postmenopausal breast, endometrial uterine, ovary, kidney, meningioma, thyroid, non-Hodgkin's lymphoma, and multiple myeloma! Furthermore, people who are overweight and who get cancer are also at higher risk of dying from the cancer.

Measuring Body Fat

There are many ways of measuring body fat. Body mass index (BMI) is a measure of adult body fat based on weight and height. It is the most commonly used, because it is easily determined and is a good proxy for assessing overall body fatness. It is not the most accurate, with dual-energy X-ray absorptiometry (DEXA) scans being one of the best, although it does require special equipment.

If you have had a bone density study, you will be familiar with this machine. It measures bone density, lean body mass, and fat. DEXA scans sometimes detect obesity in people with a normal BMI.

Another way of measuring obesity is to measure girth, or to express girth as a ratio of the hip circumference. These have the advantage of measuring abdominal fat, which some people consider more important than overall fatness. Some studies suggest that gaining weight in adulthood is more important than overall fat.

BMI   (weight in kilograms divided by height in meters squared,
         or weight in pounds x 703 divided by height in inches squared)

- Underweight   less than 18.5
- Normal   18.5–24.9
- Overweight   25–29.9
- Obese   30 or higher

Girth (waist circumference)

- Abdominal Obesity
- Men >102 cm (40 in)   Women >88 cm (35 in)

Waist-Hip Ratio (waist circumference divided by hip circumference)

- Abdominal obesity
- Men >0.9   Women >0.85

DEXA Scan (percent body fat)

- Fit   Men 14–17 percent   Women 21–24 percent
- Average   Men 18–24 percent   Women 25–31 percent
- Obese   Men 25 percent+   Women 32 percent+

The Fat Problem

Having excess body fat is a massive problem, pun intended, and a fairly recent one. Worldwide, there are about 640 million adults who are obese. This has increased by a factor of sixfold since 1980. The percentage of the world's population who are obese is 10.8 percent for men, 14.9 percent for women, and 5 percent for children, and this doesn't include those who are overweight.

There are more people in the world who are overweight or obese than who are underweight! It has been estimated that for Western countries, where the obesity problem is greatest, up to 20 percent of all cancer occurs as a result of having excess body fat. Worldwide, it results in some 4.5 million deaths each year. In particular, excess body fat is thought to account for up to 60 percent of all endometrial cancers, 36 percent of gallbladder cancers, 33 percent of kidney cancers, 17 percent of pancreatic cancers, and 11 percent of multiple myelomas.

Youth Excess Fat and Cancer

Between 1980 and 2014, overweight or obesity in children and adolescents in the US increased by more than 100 percent (from 14.7 percent to 33.4 percent of the population). There are concerns that this might be responsible for the increase in some types of cancer seen in younger people. A study using information from US state registries showed that from 1995 to 2014, the incidences of multiple myeloma, colorectal, endometrial, gallbladder, kidney, pancreas, and thyroid cancers increased in younger adults and the younger the age group, the bigger the increase in incidence. These cancers are all known to be associated with weight gain. For pancreatic cancer, excess body fat during early adulthood seems to be more important than weight gain later in life.

Assessing Body Fat and Cancer

There have been more than 1,000 studies looking at body fat and cancer risk. These are relatively easy to do, as researchers just need to have the height and weight data on a large number of people, then follow them for years and see how many get cancer. A good study, of course, needs a lot more information about other factors that could influence the results, such as smoking, diet, and physical activity.

What is more difficult research is to do an RCT of weight loss, taking a group of overweight people and get half of them to lose weight. One could then see if the number of cancers that developed over the coming years was less in that group compared to those who stayed the same weight. You can imagine the difficulties, given weight loss by dietary means is so hard to achieve, but there has been at least one large study that has done this.

A different way of doing such a study, and this has only been available since the advent and refinement of weight-loss surgery, has been to compare the cancer rates in obese groups who have, or have not, had bariatric surgery.

Excess Body Fat and Overall Cancer Risk

In 2016, the International Agency for Research into Cancer (IARC) reviewed about 1,000 epidemiological studies that looked at body fat and cancer. Most of these were observational studies, where people who were obese or overweight were compared to a group who had a normal weight, then followed to see if one group developed more cancers than the other.

The study found that the highest risk was for cancer of the uterus—endometrial, not cervical—where obese women were seven times more likely to get the disease. For esophageal cancer, there was a five times increase in risk. Lesser increases in risk were for stomach, liver, and kidney cancers, where the increase in risk was almost double, and for pancreas, meningioma, and multiple myeloma, where the risk was increased by 50 percent.

The increase in cancer risk in people with excess body fat is as follows.

• Endometrium	sevenfold (700 percent increase)
• Esophagus	fivefold (500 percent increase)
• Breast (postmenopausal)	double (100 percent increase)
• Gastric cardia	80 percent
• Liver	80 percent
• Kidney	80 percent
• Pancreas	50 percent
• Meningioma	50 percent
• Multiple myeloma	50 percent

- Colorectal   30 percent
- Gallbladder   30 percent

It has been suggested that central obesity is more important than overall obesity when it comes to cancer risk, and so perhaps it is not just fat that counts, but where it is stored in the body. Central obesity is defined as the ratio of trunk fat to peripheral fat. A group of Danish researchers investigated this by DEXA scans in nearly 6,000 older women and found those with a high proportion of central fat had a 30 percent increase in their overall risk of getting cancer.

Weight Loss and Risk Reduction

If being overweight increases the risk of getting cancer, does losing weight reverse it? Weight-loss studies through diet are notoriously difficult to undertake, but there have now been large numbers of people worldwide who have had weight-loss surgery. Most of these people lose a significant amount of weight and so form a group who can have their cancer risks compared to those obese people who have not undergone such surgery.

A study was done in Sweden where, between 1987 and 2001, obese people were recruited and offered weight-loss surgery, known as bariatric surgery. In this long-term study, 2,010 individuals chose surgery, and these were matched to a similar number who did not have surgery. At the start, the average BMI for men was 34 and for women 38, and they were followed for the next twenty years. Those who had the weight-loss surgery lost, on average, about 20 kg (44 lb). Those in the control group, who did not have surgery, did not change their weight at all.

During the years of follow-up, compared to controls, those who had the surgery had a 30 percent lower chance of dying, with fewer myocardial infarctions, diabetes, strokes, and cancer. Overall, 117 cancers occurred in those who had bariatric surgery compared to 169 in the controls, a one-third reduction. This effect was nearly all in women, with 79 women developing cancer in those who had surgery compared to 130 in the control women, a more than 40 percent reduction. The largest reduction was for endometrial cancer.

In a UK study, 8,794 obese patients underwent bariatric surgery, and a similar number of obese patients who did not were compared. Those undergoing surgery had a 77 percent overall reduction in cancer, mainly breast (75 percent reduction), endometrium (79 percent reduction), and prostate cancer (63 percent).

Colorectal Cancer

A meta-analysis of four studies found that bariatric surgery was associated with a 27 percent lower colorectal cancer risk, compared with obese nonoperated individuals.

Breast Cancer

In the WHI study, 3,460 postmenopausal women who had a normal BMI underwent DEXA scans to measure body fat. They were followed for an average of sixteen years; during this time 182 breast cancers developed. Those in the group with the highest percent fat on DEXA had double the breast cancer risk of those with the least fat, indicating that a person does not have to be overweight or obese to increase cancer risk, just have more fat.

Weight loss also benefits women who have been treated for breast cancer by preventing recurrence. In the WINS study, women previously treated for early breast cancer were randomized to change to either a low-fat diet or remained on their usual diet. Those on the low-fat diet lost almost 3 kg (6.6 lb) on average and over the follow-up period had a 24 percent reduction in the chances of their cancer recurring.

Skin Cancer

In a study of more than 4,000 obese people in Sweden, half had bariatric surgery and had a long-term weight loss of about 20 kg (44 lb), while the others did not have surgery and did not lose significant weight. After eighteen years of follow-up, those in the obesity surgery group developed twenty-three skin cancers while the others got forty-one, a more than 40 percent reduction. With melanoma, this reduction in risk was even higher, with twelve melanomas in the weight-loss group compared to twenty-nine in the control group, a more than 60 percent reduction.

Endometrial Cancer

Of all cancers, obesity is most correlated with endometrial cancer, with obese women being more than seven times more likely to develop the cancer than nonobese women. Weight loss significantly reduces this risk. In the Swedish study of bariatric surgery, women who underwent the surgery had a 46 percent lower chance of developing endometrial cancer compared to those obese women not having surgery.

How Does Excess Body Fat Cause Cancer?

Hormonal Pathways

Lipocytes, the technical name for the fat cells in our bodies, contain an enzyme called aromatase. This enzyme makes estrogen, so women with more fat have more estrogen production. Estrogen is particularly important in the development of endometrial cancer and also breast cancer in postmenopausal women.

Obese people also have lower levels of sex hormone binding globulin (SHBG) in their circulation. This protein does just that, it binds hormones so there is less available to the tissues. With a lower level, more hormone is available to stimulate hormone sensitive tissues, such as the uterus and breast, making them more prone to cancer.

Insulin and IGF-1

Body fat alters insulin metabolism, with increased insulin resistance and increased levels of insulin and insulin-like growth factor (IGF-1). These are associated with chronic inflammation and increased cancer risk.

How Much Is Too Much?

The obesity-related cancers all have a good dose response, that is, the more fat there is, the higher the risk. As a result, overweight people have a higher risk than those with a normal BMI, people who are obese have a higher risk than those overweight, and grossly obese people (BMI >40) are at the highest risk. Even in women with a normal BMI, those with more fat as measured by a DEXA scan are at increased cancer risk.

It is important to keep body fat to a minimum. The problem is that losing weight is difficult, and even if you can, maintaining the new lower weight is just as hard. It requires reduced calorie input and this involves a lot of self-control. Exercise helps a little but is not nearly as important as justifying everything that goes in the mouth.

It's said that weight control is 80 percent what you eat and 20 percent exercise. There are apps, such as MyFitnessPal, Lose It!, or SparkPeople, that are free and easy to use. They generate your body's calorie needs, and how much this needs to be reduced to meet your weight-loss goal in the timeframe you choose.

You just enter what you eat from the app database, and it shows you the number of calories and nutrients in everything you eat, in addition to daily totals. You soon learn to recognize which foods have lots of calories and should be avoided. Once you have reached your calorie limit for the day, you need to stop eating. That is the difficult part!

For those who are obese and are unable to lose weight through diet, weight-loss surgery is a definite possibility. Surgery should never be undertaken lightly, but sometimes the risks of not having surgery are worth it—think 30 percent overall mortality reduction. Gastric banding has largely been discredited as a reliable procedure for long-term weight loss, and it has been replaced by gastric sleeve or bypass procedures. An experienced surgeon with a good team of psychologists and nutritionists is essential for achieving a good outcome from bariatric surgery.

What You Should Do

- Keep body fat to a minimum.
- If you are obese and unable to lose fat by diet, consider weight-loss surgery as a means of long-term weight control.

Excess Body Fat
Decrease or Increase Risk

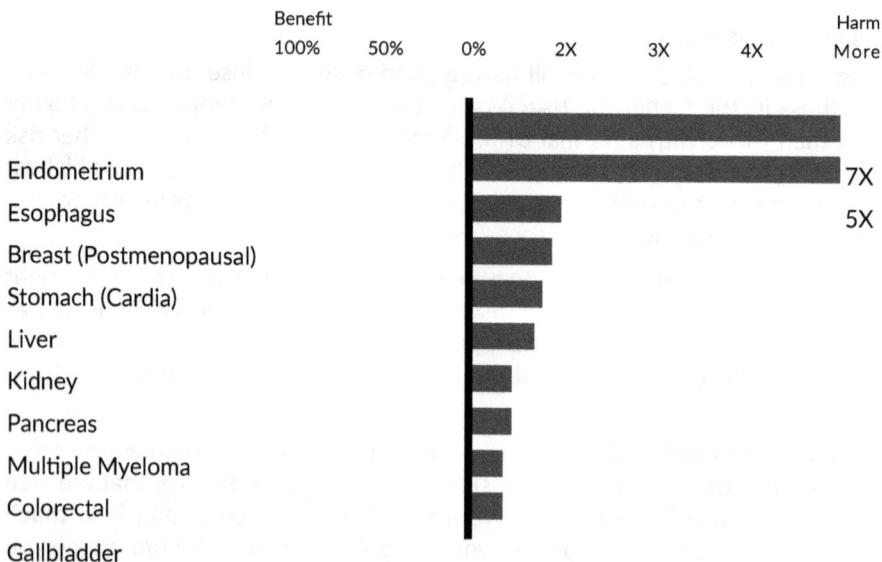

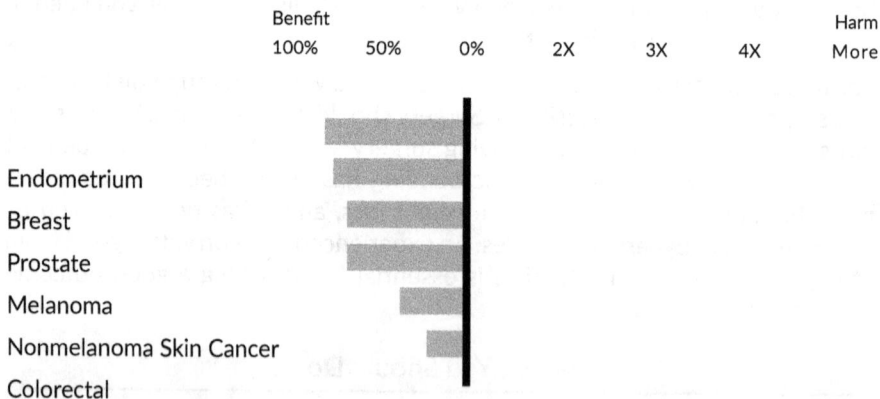

Benefit						Harm
100%	50%	0%	2X	3X	4X	More

Endometrium 7X

Esophagus 5X

Breast (Postmenopausal)

Stomach (Cardia)

Liver

Kidney

Pancreas

Multiple Myeloma

Colorectal

Gallbladder

Bariatric (Weight-Loss) Surgery in Obese People
Decrease or Increase Risk

Benefit						Harm
100%	50%	0%	2X	3X	4X	More

Endometrium

Breast

Prostate

Melanoma

Nonmelanoma Skin Cancer

Colorectal

The Gut Microbiome

What Is the Microbiome?

The microbiome is the vast number of microorganisms that exist as part of the body, largely in the gastrointestinal tract but also in the vagina and on the skin. They coexist with our own cells, and there are more cells in the microbiome than in our own body, about 110 trillion of them. For the most part, they are a variety of bacteria but there are also viruses and fungi. Most are found toward the end of the small bowel and in the colon and rectum, but there are smaller numbers throughout the gut, from mouth to anus.

The microbiome is initially acquired at birth from the mother's skin, vagina, and feces, and stabilizes about the time of weaning. Once established, it is fairly stable throughout life. The main disrupting factor is treatment with antibiotics, although dietary and lifestyle changes can also have an effect. Most of the organisms present are what we call anaerobic bacteria, with names such as *Bacteroides, Eubacterium, Bifidobacteria, Fusobacterium*, and *Peptostreptococcus*. Organisms whose names are more familiar to us, such as *Lactobacilli, Enterococcus*, and *Streptococci*, are present but are less common.

The Function of the Microbiome

This mass of organisms, the microbiome, is thought to play an important part in maintaining overall health, not just gut health. It also plays a part in developing and maintaining our immune system, our mental health, our metabolism, and our resistance to disease. Disruption has been linked to a wide range of disease from irritable bowel and inflammatory bowel disease to obesity, diabetes, and possibly cancer.

The microbiome also acts as a barrier to other organisms growing in the gut and causing disease. Antibiotic therapy disrupts this normal population of organisms in the gut. This can allow other organisms to grow, resulting in inflammation of the bowel wall leading to diarrhea.

Probiotics and Prebiotics

Probiotics. Probiotics are collections of live bacteria ingested as a way of improving health. The most common strains are *Lactobacilli* and *Bifidobacteria*, although many commercial preparations contain a much wider range of organisms. Apart from the commercial preparations, which usually come as a dried form in capsules containing billions of organisms, yogurt and other fermented foods can act like a probiotic and provide a supply of new organisms to the gut. Unfortunately, many of the organisms from these sources are destroyed by gastric acidity before they get to the lower bowel.

Prebiotics. Prebiotics are preparations of soluble fiber on which gut organisms feed and multiply, so taking a prebiotic with a probiotic is a more effective way of populating the gut with beneficial bacteria. These soluble fibers include inulin, fructose- or galactose-oligosaccharides, lactulose, and resistant fiber.

While traditionally we think of fiber as the stringy bits that stick in our teeth after eating fruits or vegetables, this fiber is completely soluble. It can be found in foods such as chicory, Jerusalem artichokes, garlic, leeks, onions, asparagus, and the outer fiber of whole grains. A typical Western diet contains little prebiotic.

This soluble fiber resists digestion, but beneficial bacteria such as Lactobacilli and Bifidobacteria feed on it and multiply, leading to a large increase in bacterial numbers and an increase in the bulk of the stools. In this process, the prebiotic is fermented and one of the products is short-chain fatty acids. These are anti-inflammatory, protect the gut lining and can benefit immunity.

Synbiotics. When taken together, the combination of probiotic and prebiotic is sometimes referred to as a synbiotic. This combination appears to be more effective at increasing the population of beneficial bacteria in the gut than either one alone.

Clinical trials of synbiotics have been done for a number of diseases and they have been shown to benefit health as a preventive measure for childhood eczema and for constipation. In patients undergoing major surgery, such as liver, pancreatic, and bowel operations, commencing synbiotics a week or more before surgery results in fewer complications, earlier return of gut function, fewer infections, and a shorter hospital stay.

Synbiotics are also used to treat inflammatory bowel disease and bowel infections, especially those such as *Clostridium difficile* infections caused by antibiotic therapy. There have been no published clinical trials as yet on their effect on cancer development.

The Microbiome and Cancer

Understanding that the microbiome plays such an important part in the body's function has only been recognized in recent years, so our knowledge is in its early stages. We still do not even know how to culture most of the organisms present in the laboratory. There have been no large human studies relating the microbiome to cancer and no large randomized trials of probiotics to see if these can prevent cancer by favorably influencing the composition of this mass of organisms.

Most of our knowledge comes from laboratory and animal studies, and much of this has been research into the relationship between the microbiome and colon, rather than other cancers. There is such a close physical relationship between the organisms and the bowel wall that this is a natural starting point. The mouse microbiome has been found to be similar to that of humans, so mice have been useful for research.

There are a number of possible ways the microbiome could influence cancer development. Several bacteria have been implicated. *Helicobacter pylori* is known to cause stomach cancer. *Bacillus fragilis*, *Escherichia coli*, and others are more common than normal in patients with colorectal cancer, but their exact role is unclear. Other possible mechanisms by which the microbiome could influence cancer development include changing the chemical content in the gut in a beneficial way by metabolizing possible carcinogens, changing the production of hormones, and improving the body's immune system.

The current state of knowledge is that we do not know if and how the microbiome affects cancer development. The situation is complicated by the relationship between what we eat and the microbiome. Are certain foods, such as red meat, causing cancer, or is it that it affects the composition of microbiome?

We will not know if influencing the composition of the microbiome can prevent cancer until there is a large randomized trial where half the participants are given a daily probiotic and prebiotic, then followed for a decade to see how many cancers develop in each group. This would need to involve tens of thousands of participants and would be a big undertaking, but it is something that could and should be done.

What You Should Do

- There is no research available yet to show that altering the microbiome can prevent cancer.

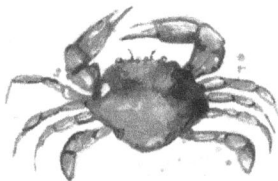

Medications to Prevent Cancer

The use of medication to prevent cancer is called chemoprevention. The idea of taking a drug to prevent a cancer that you might never get anyway, and which might have side effects, has never been popular. While few people follow this approach, those at high risk should certainly consider it.

Antiestrogens for Breast Cancer

Taking an antiestrogen for five years can result in a major reduction in the chances of getting breast cancer. About 80 percent of breast cancers are what we call estrogen receptor positive, that is, they need estrogen to grow. If deprived of estrogen, they will not develop, or if already present, will often shrivel away, and so these drugs are an important part of treating breast cancer.

The original drugs developed for this purpose were tamoxifen, which blocks the uptake of estrogen into breast cells and breast cancer cells, and a group of drugs called aromatase inhibitors (AIs) that lower estrogen levels in postmenopausal women by reducing the body's production of estrogen.

They have been used for decades and trials have shown that they are effective in the treatment of breast cancer, and they also greatly reduce the chances of developing breast cancer in otherwise well but high-risk women. They are a true preventive agent. Studies have shown that high-risk women who take these for five or more years can halve their chances of getting breast cancer, and the benefit can last long after the antiestrogen has been ceased.

Some women are put off by the side effects. Tamoxifen can aggravate or bring on menopausal hot flashes, and it increases a woman's risk of getting uterine cancer (not if she has had a hysterectomy or is taking a progestin), while aromatase inhibitors aggravate hot flashes and can cause muscle and joint pains.

There is a new generation of drugs called selective estrogen receptor modulators (SERMs). These were developed to prevent osteoporosis and in many ways are similar to tamoxifen, which was a first-generation SERM. The advantage of them is that they are even more effective at preventing breast cancer than tamoxifen or AIs. They also help prevent the osteoporosis and vaginal atrophy that occurs after menopause, and they do not cause uterine cancer. They appear to be virtually side-effect free. The best drugs are lasofoxifene and raloxifene, with lasofoxifene having an 80 percent reduction in breast cancer occurrence and with no more side effects than a placebo.

The Oral Contraceptive Pill for Ovarian Cancer

While preventing ovarian cancer is not, in itself, a good reason for taking the oral contraceptive pill (OCP), many women take it for contraception. A side benefit is a considerably reduced chance of getting ovarian cancer. Virtually every study that has looked at this comes to the same conclusion. It is estimated that for every five years of OCP use, the risk of getting ovarian cancer reduces by 20 percent, so that women who have taken the "pill" for fifteen years have at least halved their chances of getting the disease. This protective effect lasts long after stopping the OCP, and there is still some benefit twenty years later.

Antiandrogens for Prostate Cancer

Because prostate cancer is so common in Western populations, it is not surprising that there have been trials of drug therapy to try to prevent the disease. As with using drugs to prevent breast cancer, the basic approach is to try to change the hormonal environment, in this case androgens, rather than estrogens as in breast cancer. A group of drugs called 5-alpha-reductase inhibitors block the production of androgens. In clinical trials they can reduce the occurrence of prostate cancer by 25–30 percent. They seem to mainly prevent the less aggressive forms of prostate cancer.

Aspirin

Long-term use of low-dose aspirin has been shown to reduce the chances of dying from a number of different cancers. Over 130,000 people enrolled in the Nurses' Health Study and the Health Professionals Follow-up Study were followed for thirty-two years. Aspirin use was recorded at the start and every two years thereafter.

During the follow-up period, 8,271 women and 4,591 men died of cancer. Overall, women who used aspirin had a 7 percent lower chance of dying from cancer, and for men, this was 15 percent. Only low-dose aspirin was needed to be effective, and it had to be continued for at least six years. For specific cancer types, there was a 30 percent lower risk of dying from colorectal cancer, an 11 percent lower risk from breast cancer, a 23 percent lower risk from prostate cancer, and a 14 percent lower risk from lung cancer in men.

A cohort study using data from 12,969,400 participants in the Korean National Health Information Database found that the use of low-dose aspirin for at least five years, and especially if used for nine or more years, was associated with a reduction in lung cancer. For those who used it for nine or more years, there was a 10 percent lower lung cancer risk.

Other studies have also shown that long-term low-dose aspirin reduces the incidence of hepatocellular cancer of the liver (49 percent reduction), ovarian cancer (23 percent lower), lung cancer (20 percent), malignant melanoma (20 percent), breast cancer (16 percent), and colonic polyps and colorectal cancer

(16–30 percent). Even patients with a genetic predisposition to bowel cancer, such as Lynch syndrome, can significantly reduce their chances of getting cancer by taking aspirin.

It is important to note that these benefits are from low-dose aspirin, and it needs to be taken for at least five years to see any benefit. It seems to be the antiplatelet function of aspirin, rather than the anti-inflammatory action that provides the benefit. Taking nonsteroidal anti-inflammatory drugs does not seem to have the same effect.

Low-dose aspirin is, for the most part, a safe drug and its only significant side effect is to slightly increase the risk of bleeding by making platelets less sticky. In contrast to the evidence above, some RCTs of aspirin have questioned the benefits of taking aspirin as a preventive measure, given the small but real increased risk of having a bleed into the brain resulting in a stroke.

Statins

A number of studies have indicated that people who take statins to control their cholesterol have a 37 percent decrease in their risk of getting hepatocellular cancer. These studies were combined into one large meta-analysis with a total of 1.6 million people in multiple countries, so it is likely this is a real effect. The benefit seems to be mostly in East Asian people with hepatitis B infections.

What You Should Do

- If at high risk for colorectal cancer, consider low-dose aspirin (80–100 mg) daily unless concerned about bleeding.
- If at high risk for breast cancer, consider taking a SERM, such as raloxifene or lasofoxifene.

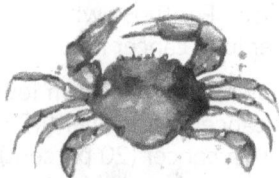

Pesticides and Herbicides

In 2015, the International Agency for Research on Cancer (IARC) classified some of the commonly used agricultural chemicals as carcinogenic: malathion for prostate cancer; diazinon for lung cancer; and glyphosate, malathion, and diazinon for non-Hodgkin's lymphoma. Most of these agricultural chemicals reach us through consumption of fruits and vegetables, where they are used to keep insects and weeds under control. In the US more than 90 percent of the population have detectable pesticides in their urine and blood. Organic foods that are grown without herbicides and pesticides are less likely to contain chemical residues than nonorganic foods.

In the NutriNet-Santé study from France, a Web-based cohort study, 68,946 study participants reported on their consumption of organic foods. They were followed for five years and 1,340 cancers developed. Those who had the highest consumption of organic foods had a 25 percent lower chance of getting cancer, compared to those who ate the least organic foods. The benefits were for postmenopausal breast cancer and non-Hodgkin's lymphoma.

In another study, the Million Women Study from the UK, 623,080 women reported their frequency of eating organic foods; 7 percent said they usually or always ate organic. After seven years of follow-up, 53,769 cancers had developed. Compared to women who never ate organic, the women who reported usually or always eating organic had a 21 percent lower chance of getting non-Hodgkin's lymphoma. There was no benefit for breast cancer, nor for any other cancer.

What You Should Do

- Avoid contact with herbicides and pesticides, and where possible buy organically grown foods.

Organic Diets, Pesticides, and Herbicides

Decrease or Increase Risk

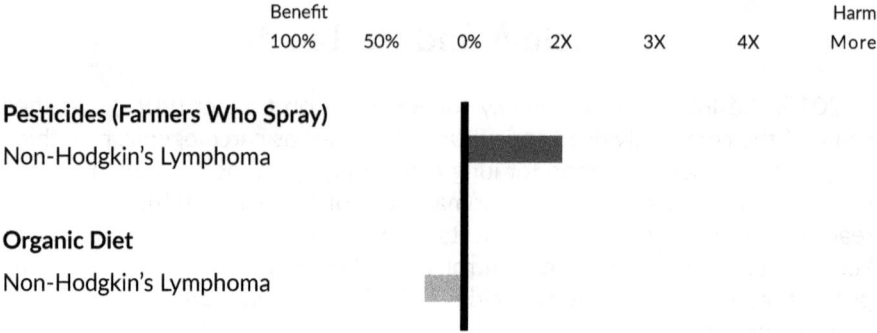

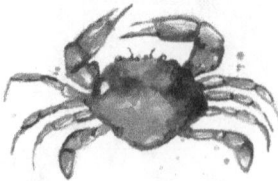

	Benefit						Harm
	100%	50%	0%	2X	3X	4X	More

Pesticides (Farmers Who Spray)

Non-Hodgkin's Lymphoma

Organic Diet

Non-Hodgkin's Lymphoma

Physical Activity

What Is Physical Activity?

Physical activity can take many forms: from low-level activities, like walking and gardening, to a job that requires a lot of movement, to higher-intensity exercises, such as running and weight training, to intense-exercise regimes, such as triathlon or marathon training.

Apart from the intensity, there are other factors to be considered when assessing exercise. Some exercise is classified as aerobic: where the aim is primarily improving cardiac and respiratory function and calorie burning. Others are categorized as resistance training, where the aim is to improve muscle strength and size. In reality, there is overlap between the two.

Another factor to be taken into consideration is the duration of physical activity: how does the physical activity of a cleaner, who works eight hours a day but does no intentional exercise outside of work, compare to an office worker, who runs for an hour each day but sits for the rest of the day?

Measuring Physical Activity

There is a standard measure of physical activity, the MET. This stands for metabolic equivalent of task. It is the rate of energy expenditure for that person's weight as compared to their energy expended by sitting quietly (the basal metabolic rate or BMR). For example, sitting quietly or sleeping has a MET of 1, while a sprint has a MET of over 15, so sprinting uses fifteen times the energy of sitting.

To make allowance for the duration of exercise and the number of times each week physical activity is undertaken, total physical activity is measured as MET hours per week. When researching how physical activity affects health, a standard measure is essential to allow for all the different forms of exercise. Some examples of METs for different activities are shown here, although the figures for any particular activity will vary with the intensity of the activity and the person's weight.

Activity	MET
• Slow walk	2.5
• Yoga	2.5
• Gardening	4

- Golf   4.5
- Dancing   4.8
- Fast walk   5
- Lifting weights   6
- Swimming   8
- Boot camp   8
- Playing soccer   10
- Fast run   11

Physical Activity and Body Fat

A further factor to be considered when looking at physical activity and health is its relationship to body fat. Undertaking physical activity increases muscle, and any increase in muscle is often at the expense of body fat. Two people might have the same BMI, but the physically active person will have more muscle and less body fat than the inactive person.

There is evidence that shows that physically active people have a lower cancer risk. We also know that excess body fat increases cancer risk. Is it the physical activity itself that is the beneficial factor, or is it because these people have less body fat? These factors can be difficult to separate when undertaking research into physical activity and cancer, but in general, it is believed that being physically active does provide benefit over and above that from any reduction in body fat.

How Can Physical Activity Reduce Cancer Risk?

Physical activity, apart from reducing body fat, has a wide range of beneficial effects on the body. In particular, physical activity reduces insulin sensitivity and reduces circulating IGF-1 levels. These are known to increase risk for a number of cancers. Physical activity also improves the body's immune function, and this should reduce tumor development. Finally, physical activity lowers the levels of circulating estrogens, and this will reduce the development of postmenopausal breast cancer and uterine cancer.

Physical Activity and Cancer

The reduction in cancer risk from physical activity is seen for a variety of cancers, including colon, breast, uterine, endometrium, liver, pancreas, and stomach cancers.

For colon cancer, four meta-analyses have pooled the results of smaller studies and have shown that the most physically active people have a 15–25 percent lower chance of developing colon cancer compared to the least active. This does not seem to apply to cancer in the lowest part of the large bowel, the rectum.

For breast cancer, meta-analyses have shown that the most physically active postmenopausal women reduce their breast cancer risk by 13 percent compared to the least active. For premenopausal women, the benefit is a 7 percent reduction. One analysis determined that for every ten MET hours/week of exercise, postmenopausal breast cancer risk diminished by 2 percent. Analysis of vigorous physical exercise, as opposed to the total activity, showed that for every thirty minutes of vigorous exercise per day, breast cancer risk was reduced by 7–9 percent, and this was for both premenopausal and postmenopausal women.

A study of 110,599 teachers in California recorded information on their physical activity from their high school years until the start of the study—2,649 were subsequently diagnosed with invasive breast cancer and 593 with in situ (noninvasive) breast cancer. In this study, long-term strenuous activity was associated with a 20 percent lower risk of invasive breast cancer and a 30 percent lower risk of in situ cancer. This reduction in cancer was predominantly for hormone-receptor negative cancers, a more aggressive type of breast cancer. The group with the most benefit was those who did long-term strenuous activity of more than five hours per week.

Meta-analyses of studies of endometrial cancer found that increased physical activity was associated with a reduction in incidence. This applied to recreational activity, occupational activity, and walking and cycling.

A Japanese study followed 79,771 men and women, investigating the effect of all forms of physical activity on cancer development, and this included both sport and occupational activity. During the follow-up, 4,334 cancers developed. Overall, men who were the most active had a 13 percent reduction in cancer compared to the least active men, and for women the cancer reduction was 16 percent. Significant reductions occurred in colon cancer, liver cancer, pancreatic and stomach cancers, and for these particular cancers, the reduction in risk was about 40 percent.

How Much Is Enough?

There are no consistent guidelines on how much exercise you should do to prevent cancer but, in general, more is better. A good guide comes from the Nurses' Health Study where women who did twenty-one MET hours/week, which equates to about seven hours of brisk walking each week, had half the number of colon cancers compared to those who only did two MET hours/week, about a one-hour slow walk each week. There are numerous apps available to help you keep track of your physical activity. You can also use wearable devices, such as a Fitbit.

What You Should Do

- Exercise regularly, in whatever form you can manage, preferably daily. Try for a minimum of twenty MET hours/week. That is roughly an hour's brisk walk each day.

Physical Activity

Decrease or Increase Risk

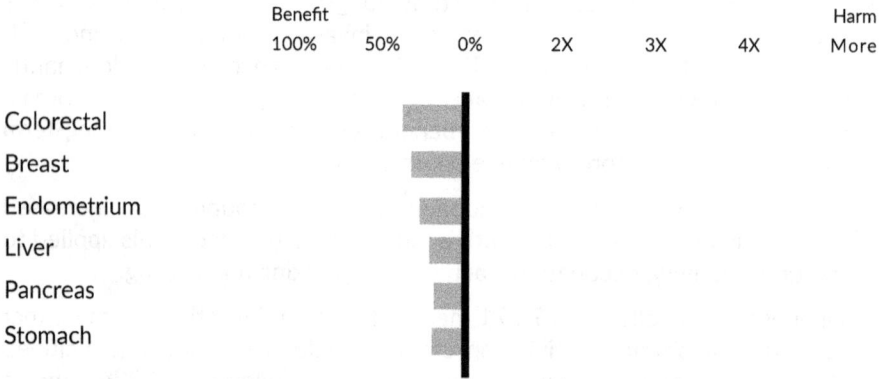

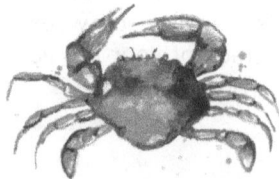

Benefit						Harm
100%	50%	0%	2X	3X	4X	More

Colorectal

Breast

Endometrium

Liver

Pancreas

Stomach

Preventive Surgery

It seems a radical approach to remove an organ just because it might develop a cancer at some stage, but for some people the risk of cancer is so high that it is worth it.

Bilateral Mastectomies to Prevent Breast Cancer

The two major breast cancer-causing genetic mutations, BRCA1 and BRCA2, are not rare. It has been estimated that about 1 in 400 women will have one of these mutations, and it's higher in Ashkenazi Jews (of Eastern European descent). Women who have one of these mutations have a 70 percent chance of developing breast cancer at some stage in their lives, and this is usually at a young age. They also have a 40 percent chance of developing ovarian cancer, although this usually occurs a little later in life. Testing for these genetic mutations is relatively straightforward, and anyone with a strong family history of breast cancer, especially if it occurred at a young age or if there is ovarian cancer in the family, should do it.

With such a high risk, it is not surprising that these women often choose preventive surgery in the form of bilateral mastectomies, often combined with breast reconstructions. Most people would see this as preferable to risk getting breast cancer, then needing surgery, chemotherapy, radiation therapy, and even then, still having a chance of dying from the disease. Angelina Jolie was in many ways a pioneer and example to young women by having this done. It is major surgery and the end result is rarely perfect, but some choose it for the peace of mind and knowledge that they have done everything they can to stop getting breast cancer.

The surgery can only remove at most 95 percent of breast tissue. Breast tissue extends through to the skin, around into the armpit, and in some people even down the arm a short distance. Some women even have a rudimentary nipple in the armpit and after childbirth this can leak milk. Without an extensive excision of all the skin and the tissue in the armpit, it is not possible to surgically remove all breast tissue, and to do so would be disfiguring. Despite this, prophylactic mastectomies still result in a major reduction in breast cancer risk.

Ovarian and Tubal Surgery to Prevent Ovarian Cancer

Removing the fallopian tubes and ovaries protects against ovarian cancer. This is called bilateral salpingo-oophorectomy (BSO). It reduces the chances of getting this cancer by 80 percent. This surgery is common for endometriosis or cysts, and even having one ovary removed reduces the overall cancer risk. For someone who has inherited the BRCA1 genetic mutation, there is almost a one in two chance of developing ovarian cancer, and almost a one in four chance for BRCA2.

With such a high risk of developing what is often a fatal cancer, most women with these mutations have BSO surgery once they have finished having children, then go on hormone replacement to make up for the reduced hormone production. Such surgery is often keyhole, minimally invasive, and a day's stay in the hospital. It is important that the fallopian tubes are removed and as well as the ovaries, as these can sometimes be a source of ovarian cancer.

Removing Undescended Testes to Prevent Testicular Cancer

The testes develop inside the abdomen. About the time of birth, they descend into the scrotum. In about 1 percent of boys, this descent does not take place, and one or both testes can arrest anywhere from the kidney to the groin. This is called undescended testicles or cryptorchidism. In most cases, they arrest in the groin and surgery is usually successful in bringing them the rest of the way into the scrotum. Failure to enter the scrotum results in infertility, and the undescended testes are also at increased risk of cancer.

Men born with undescended testes have a more than five-fold increase in their chance of developing testicular cancer, usually in their thirties and forties. Consideration should be given to removing the undescended testicles to remove the cancer risk, and this can be done by minimally invasive keyhole surgery. There is little point in keeping it as it is nonfunctioning from a fertility point of view.

Total Colectomy to Prevent Colorectal Cancer

For some people, the best way to prevent colorectal cancer is to remove as much of the large bowel as possible. This is major surgery with significant risk of complications from the surgery; living without a large bowel is not easy. At best, it involves creating a pouch out of the small bowel and fixing this to the anus. This might sound reasonable, but the result is frequent, watery bowel actions as the colon is not present to absorb the fluid from the contents.

At worst, the surgery results in a permanent stoma with the end of the small bowel being brought to the surface of the body, called an ileostomy, and the person wears a bag to collect the effluent. However, if you have a condition where it means you will almost certainly get colorectal cancer when young, and possibly die from cancer spread, it might be the best option. Situations where this occurs are the inherited familial adenomatous polyposis syndrome (FAP) or someone with long-standing ulcerative colitis involving the whole colon, as these people also have a high risk of getting colorectal cancer.

What You Should Do

- If you have inherited a genetic mutation, which puts you at high risk of developing cancer at a young age, consider preventive surgery to minimize the risk.

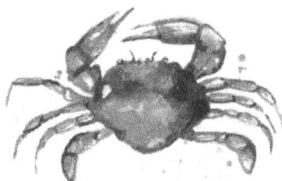

Radiation

What Is Radiation?

Radiation is the movement of energy, usually in the form of waves but it can be subatomic-sized particles. We normally think of radiation as traveling through the air, but some forms of radiation can travel through space or even solid materials. The denser the material through which the radiation is traveling, the quicker the energy is absorbed. That is why rooms where X-rays are taken have lead shielding in the walls.

There is a wide range of types of radiation, and they are usually grouped by the amount of energy they carry.

Examples include high energy radiation, often called ionizing radiation.

- Alpha, beta, or gamma radiation from radioactive isotopes
- X-rays created by radiograph machines and computed tomography (CT) scanners
- Neutrons that travel as cosmic rays from space.

These high-energy types of radiation can be dangerous, as the energy they carry is sufficient to break an electron from an atom, a process called ionization. These loose electrons can damage DNA and so lead to cancer. Researcher and physicist/chemist Marie Curie, who won a Nobel Prize in Physics for her pioneering work in radiation in 1903, died from aplastic anemia, a cancer-related disease, from exposure to radiation. She was exposed to a lot of radiation during her lifetime as the dangers of radiation were not well understood at that time. She often carried radioactive material in her pocket!

Lower energy types of radiation include the following.

- Ultraviolet (UV) radiation, which still has enough energy to damage the DNA in cells.
- Visible light
- Infrared radiation
- Microwaves
- Radio waves, such as from cell phones and power transmission lines
- Acoustic radiation, such as sound or ultrasound

These lower energy forms of radiation dissipate their energy in the material through which they are passing, sometimes causing heat.

Ionizing Radiation

How Does Ionizing Radiation Cause Cancer?

Massive doses of radiation to the body are usually fatal, through burns and internal organ failure. This occurred in those people closest to the center of the atomic bombings of Hiroshima and Nagasaki during World War II, or in workers at the Chernobyl nuclear accident in 1986.

Lesser doses can cause cancer, often many years later. For example, after the Chernobyl disaster, a cloud of nuclear waste containing radioactive isotopes, including radioactive iodine (I-131), was blown downwind and settled on the land. Cows ate the contaminated grass and some of the isotopes collected in the milk.

The body concentrates iodine in the thyroid gland, as it is needed for thyroxine production. Children who drank the milk were more likely to get thyroid cancer as a result of excessive radiation from the I-131. The most common cancer caused by radiation is leukemia. The blood-producing bone marrow is the most active of all tissues, and so is most susceptible to radiation damage.

Ionizing radiation damages the DNA in cells and in particular it affects those cells that are dividing. Cells try to reverse this damage, but often it is irreversible. Badly damaged cells die, but those that survive can have incorrectly repaired genetic material in them, so the genes do not function normally.

This can lead to abnormal growth and cancer. In particular, if a tumor-suppressor gene is damaged, the cancer risk is much higher. Leukemia would normally appear two to ten years after the radiation, but cancer of solid organs might not appear for more than ten years, and up to forty years later.

The effect of radiation received by the body is cumulative, so that over a lifetime, the damage done by radiation gradually builds up. This makes repeated exposure dangerous, and the cells of growing children are particularly at risk.

Sources of Ionizing Radiation

Natural Radiation

Most of the ionizing radiation to which we are exposed comes from natural sources. The amount of radiation we are exposed to over a lifetime from natural sources is about four times the amount we get from artificial sources, such as diagnostic X-rays. With the increasing use of computed tomography (CT) scans, this gap is rapidly narrowing. In the US, it is estimated that radiation from diagnostic tests now equals that from natural sources.

Radon Gas. One natural source is radon, a naturally occurring radioactive gas that occurs from the decay of thorium, radium, and uranium, normal elements in the earth's crust. They are more common in some parts of the world than others. Radon gas is known to accumulate in poorly ventilated buildings, where it has come from the building materials. After smoking, naturally occurring radon is the second most common cause of lung cancer, as it is inhaled as a gas.

Cosmic Radiation. The other main natural source of radiation to which we are exposed is cosmic radiation. These are mainly protons emitted by the sun, and they also come from deep space, probably the remnants of supernovae. This radiation reacts with atoms in the atmosphere to create a shower of X-rays, protons, alpha particles, electrons, and neutrons—all forms of radiation.

For most of us, this is a tiny dose, and it is something with which organisms have existed from the beginning of their evolution. However, some areas have a higher exposure than others, depending on the earth's magnetic field and the height above sea level.

People living at high altitudes can have twice the exposure of people at sea level. This is a particular problem for airline crew, frequent flyers, and astronauts who get about five times the annual radiation exposure of a worker at a nuclear plant! Even so, a pilot's cancer risk is only about 0.5 percent higher than everyone else. You would have to fly for thirty hours to get the same amount of radiation as you would from one chest X-ray.

Diagnostic and Therapeutic Radiation

It seems strange that, on one hand, radiation can cause cancer, yet, on the other hand, it can be used to treat cancer. The difference is the dose. Tiny doses do little harm, higher doses can predispose to cancer, and high doses kill cancer cells.

Therapeutic Radiation. The therapeutic radiation used to treat cancer has such an intense dose that the cancer cells are killed by the radiation. Normal cells are also irradiated in this process, but cells that are dividing, such as cancer cells, are more susceptible to the radiation. Normal cells, for example, the skin through which the radiation travels to get to the cancer being treated, are damaged to some extent but the dose of radiation is carefully calculated so that it is enough to kill cancer, but not normal tissue.

New techniques have been developed, so that the normal tissues get a minimum dose, such as pinpointing the X-ray beam by CT guidance or focusing the beam from multiple points directly onto the tumor being treated. A rare side effect of therapeutic radiation comes from around the edge of the beam, where there is some scatter of the X-rays. As a result, the tissues just beyond the area being treated can incidentally receive a lower dose.

In certain circumstances, this lower dose can predispose to cancer. Hodgkin's lymphoma is a lymphatic cancer that tends to occur in childhood and young adults. Treatment might involve directing radiation to the lymph nodes inside the chest. In this situation, the scatter from the treatment can extend onto the inner breast. So, women having this treatment are at a higher risk of getting breast cancer in the inner breast many years later.

Diagnostic Radiation. Diagnostic radiation comes from the X-rays received during a radiograph, during a CT scan, or from an isotope injected as part of a nuclear scan. The dose used to get an image is much smaller than that used to treat cancer, and for many forms of imaging it can be regarded as harmless. Tests like a chest X-ray, a bone X-ray, or a mammogram all have minimal doses.

However, some tests have a higher dose, and this can be a concern from a cancer risk point of view. This is more worrying if the person having the test is young, as young tissues are more susceptible to radiation damage, or if the test is being repeated on a number of occasions. As already mentioned, any damage from the radiation received on each occasion accumulates in the body.

Different diagnostic tests with their dose in milliSievert (mSv) include the following.

• DEXA scan (bone density)	0.001 mSv
• Foot or similar X-ray	0.001 mSv
• Dental X-ray	0.005 mSv
• Chest X-ray	0.1 mSv
• Mammogram	0.4 mSv
• CT head	2 mSv
• Isotope lung or bone scan	2–4 mSv
• CT for coronary calcium score	3 mSv
• CT chest or abdomen	7–10 mSv
• PET scan	25 mSv

A CT scan results in the body receiving 100 to 250 times the radiation of a conventional X-ray. People who are overweight require a higher dose to get good quality films, and often scans with and without an injection of contrast material are taken during the same examination, all of which increases the radiation exposure. Older machines generally give more radiation exposure than newer CT scanners. Repeat scans, even years apart, add to the total radiation damage.

The Cancer Risk from Diagnostic Radiation

Because it is not ethically possible to carry out human trials on radiation exposure and the subsequent development of cancer, our knowledge of cancer risks from radiation come from populations who have been incidentally exposed to radiation. They are followed for many years to see if they develop more cancers than would normally be expected.

The group most studied are the survivors of the atomic bombs dropped on Hiroshima and Nagasaki during World War II. More than 100,000 survivors had their radiation exposure estimated by the distance they were from the explosion center and have been followed for sixty years. It was found that the greater the exposure and the younger their age at the time, the greater the risk of developing a future cancer. It has been argued that this is not relevant to diagnostic radiation, as the doses, even from multiple CT scans, are much lower than those received by the atomic blast victims. It is worth noting, however, that even those distant from the blast and who only got a small amount of radiation still had a slightly higher cancer risk.

A study from Australia looked at the cancer risk in 680,000 young people who had CT scans done between the ages of one and nineteen. It compared their rate of cancer development over the next ten years to the Australian population in the same age group. Over this ten years, 3,150 cancers developed in those who had a CT scan in childhood.

Overall, children who had a CT scan were 24 percent more likely to get a cancer, and the risk increased by 16 percent for each additional CT scan. The risks were also higher the younger the age at first scan, with a 35 percent increase in risk in those scanned at ages one to four. The CT scans in this study were all done prior to 2005. Modern CT scan machines do give a lower dose, nevertheless, the message is that children should not have a CT scan unless absolutely necessary.

One risk model has suggested that for every 1,000 people having a 10 mSv CT scan, such as abdomen or chest, one person will develop cancer as a result of that scan at some stage in their life. This risk is said to increase to 1 in 500–600 if the CT scan is performed before age twenty. For most people, the cancer risk from diagnostic radiation is minimal, and the benefits from having an X-ray or scan usually far outweigh any risk. But be wary of unnecessary or excessive numbers of CT scans.

What You Should Do

Question the need for a CT scan if—

- There does not seem to be a good reason to have it.
- There is some other diagnostic test that does not involve radiation and which will give the same result, such as an ultrasound or a magnetic resonance imaging (MRI).
- The person having the scan is young.
- If the person has already had a lot of CT scans.

Ionizing Radiation

Decrease or Increase Risk

Benefit						Harm
100%	50%	0%	2X	3X	4X	More

CT Scan in Childhood

Any cancer

Ultraviolet Radiation (UV)

Apart from natural ionizing radiation, the only time you are likely to encounter ionizing radiation is when you need some sort of diagnostic imaging. On the other hand, you get UV radiation every time you go outside during daylight hours.

The difference is that ionizing radiation is high in energy and so even short bursts, such as a CT scan, can do damage to DNA. UV radiation has much lower energy. It can still damage DNA, but because of its lower energy, it needs longer exposure to cause harm.

While X-rays and gamma rays can penetrate deep into the body, UV radiation only affects the skin. In particular, ultraviolet B (UVB) (responsible for sunburns) result in DNA damage to the skin cells and so makes them more prone to cancer. Ultraviolet A (UVA), which penetrate further into the skin to cause premature aging, and as well as UVB, can both release free oxygen radicals. This oxidative process can also damage DNA.

Preventing UV exposure is dealt with in detail in the chapter on "Skin Cancer." Information about the benefits of UV sunlight is found in the section on vitamin D located in the chapter on "Vitamins and Minerals."

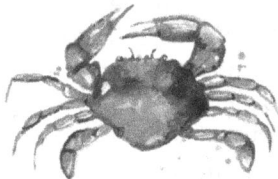

Smoking

There is no doubt that tobacco use causes cancer, and even people who live with a smoker and breathe secondhand smoke have an increased cancer risk.

How Does Smoking Cause Cancer?

Tobacco smoke has been shown to contain at least fifty different carcinogens, chemicals that can cause cancer. On inhaling the smoke, these chemicals come into contact with the lining of the breathing passages and lungs and damage these cells. Some of these chemicals are absorbed into the blood, so are carried around the body, where they can also cause harm. Regardless of the source, cigarettes, cigars, or a pipe, tobacco smoke is still inhaled together with these carcinogens. Tobacco can also be chewed or inhaled as snuff, and carcinogens are absorbed into the body.

A wide variety of carcinogens have been identified but some of the most significant are nitrosamines, polycyclic aromatic hydrocarbons, radioactive polonium, and benzene. These chemicals are found in the tar component of the smoke—what is left after the nicotine and water have been removed. The amount of carcinogen does vary with the type of tobacco used, and if there is a filter on the cigarette.

Smokers of high-tar cigarettes have a higher mortality than smokers of low-tar cigarettes. When a cigarette is inhaled, 80 percent of the particles inhaled are deposited on the lining of the respiratory tract and not exhaled. Smoke from a burning cigarette that is not inhaled contains more carcinogens, as it has not been through the filter, but it is diluted by the surrounding air, so overall is not as harmful. Passive smoking results in a mixture of this smoke and exhaled filtered smoke being inhaled.

Not all these inhaled carcinogens do damage. Some are deactivated by the body's defense mechanisms, such as antioxidants, but many are not deactivated and can damage DNA. This DNA damage might be repaired by the body so no harm is done, but often the DNA damage is unrepaired. This damage to DNA can be to genes that regulate cell growth. For example, the mutations resulting from the DNA damage can activate oncogenes that stimulates cell growth or deactivate tumor-suppressor genes that prevent the controlled death of rogue cells. As a result, uncontrolled cell growth can occur and this is cancer.

Other factors can influence the effect of these inhaled and absorbed carcinogens. Fruits and vegetables contain antioxidants, and these can help deactivate the inhaled carcinogens, so people who eat these get less smoking-related cancers. On the other hand, alcohol has the opposite effect and seems to work synergistically with the tobacco carcinogens to increase cancer risk in people who both smoke and drink. Other factors that multiply the cancer effect of tobacco include asbestos dust inhalation, silica dust inhalation, and radon gas inhalation, such as in uranium mine workers.

Tobacco smoking can also damage the immune system and increases the risk of both infections and cancer.

What Cancers Are Caused by Smoking?

Tobacco use has been proven to be a cause of cancers of the respiratory tract and lung, kidney, bladder, oral cavity, esophagus, stomach, and pancreas. There are other cancers that are linked to tobacco use but the association is not so strong. These include myeloid leukemia, liver cancer, gallbladder cancer, and childhood cancers. Cancers of the breast, ovary, prostate, brain, and skin, including melanoma, are unlikely to be caused by smoking. Women who smoke get less cancer of the endometrium of the uterus.

Respiratory Tract and Lung Cancer. Smoking accounts for 85 percent of squamous cancers of the lung in men, and about 50 percent of them in women. For cancer of the larynx in the upper respiratory tract, smoking causes 65 percent of cancers in men and 25 percent in women. The cancer risk is fifteen times that of a nonsmoker.

A nonsmoker has about a one in seventy chance of developing lung cancer, a current smoker has a one in six chance, and if they have been a heavy smoker for thirty years or more, this rises to one in three. This risk sharply declines after quitting, with the risk dropping to one in thirty for someone who stopped twenty years ago. Passive smoking also causes respiratory cancers.

Bladder and Kidney Cancer. Smokers have three times the likelihood of developing bladder cancer compared to nonsmokers, and it accounts for more than one-third of all cases of these cancers in men, and one in seven cases in women. For kidney cancer, the risk is slightly lower, and for both, the risk reduces once a person quits.

Some carcinogens from smoking are excreted through the kidneys and so can damage the cells of the renal tract. The risk is lower in the kidney, because urine passes through quickly, but urine is stored in the bladder so there is longer contact of the carcinogens with the bladder lining cells.

Gastrointestinal Tract Cancer. Oral cavity cancer, squamous cancer of the esophagus, and pancreatic cancer occur at three to five times the rate in these organs in smokers, compared to nonsmokers. Tobacco use accounts for almost 50 percent of all cases of squamous cancer of the esophagus, 40 percent of oral cavity cancer, and 25 percent of all pancreatic cancers.

It does increase the risk of stomach cancer but at a lower level of risk. Again, the risk decreases in those who quit. There is direct contact of the lining of the mouth with carcinogens from tobacco, some of these are swallowed so they can affect the lining of the esophagus and the stomach.

Uterine Endometrium. Smokers have about half the chance of getting cancer of the endometrium compared to nonsmokers. This is thought to be due to an antiestrogen effect.

What You Should Do

- If you are a smoker, quit now, as this has been shown to significantly reduce the cancer risks from smoking.
- If you live with a smoker, insist on them not smoking in enclosed spaces where you might inhale the secondhand smoke.
- If you do not smoke, do not start!

Smoking

Decrease or Increase Risk

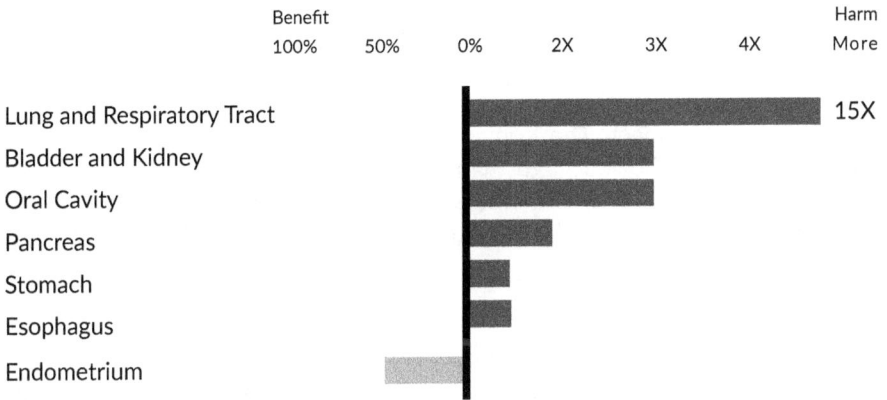

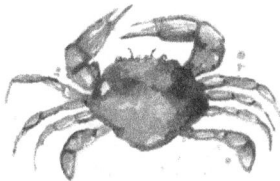

Benefit						Harm
100%	50%	0%	2X	3X	4X	More

Lung and Respiratory Tract · · · 15X
Bladder and Kidney
Oral Cavity
Pancreas
Stomach
Esophagus
Endometrium

Stress and Cancer

There is nothing new about the concept that the mind might influence the development of cancer. The Roman physician and philosopher, Galen, who lived more than 2,000 years ago, made the observation that breast cancer was more common in "melancholic" women than in "sanguine" women. We are still trying to figure this out, and many hundreds of research studies later there is still not complete consensus.

What Is Stress?

While we are generally aware when we are stressed and the cause might be obvious, few of us understand what is going on in our bodies to make us feel this way. Normally, to become stressed we need two things to happen. First, there must be some event to precipitate the stress, and second, we must perceive this as disturbing enough to cause some degree of distress, even if only subconsciously.

Measuring Stress

As indicated above, there are two components to stress, the event and the response. Measuring the event is relatively easy and there are tables that put a numerical value on stressful life events. One of the most commonly used is the Holmes-Rahe Stress Inventory, where the score varies from 11 to 100.

Some examples include these.

- Death of spouse   100
- Marital separation   65
- Major injury or illness   53
- Pregnancy   40
- Changing jobs   36
- Child leaving home   29
- Problems at work   23
- Change in sleeping habits   16
- Vacation   13
- Parking ticket   11

The scores from events can be added up for a period of time, say the last five years, and this can provide a measure for stressful events over a period leading up to a diagnosis of cancer. Of course, this scoring might not fully apply to everyone. Some might regard a pregnancy as not at all stressful, while a family vacation could be highly stressful, but it does allow a standardized scoring system. There are a number of other similar scoring systems.

A more difficult task is to assess how any individual responds to an event. We all know people who are "highly stressed" and do not seem to cope with even a minor readjustment to their lives, while we know others who are "chilled" and nothing seems to bother them. This measurement is a psychological assessment that focuses on the individual's subjective evaluation of their ability to cope with a specific event. A common measure is the Perceived Stress Scale, which is a measure of the degree to which situations in life are appraised as stressful.

How Stress Might Cause Cancer

During periods of stress, physical and chemical changes occur in the body. The response in the brain triggers the release of neurotransmitters, such as adrenaline, serotonin, and dopamine; and hormones, such as cortisol, ACTH, and prolactin. These can suppress the immune system, which in a chronic or recurrent situation could possibly lead to an increased risk of cancer developing.

Stress and Cancer

Research into stress and cancer requires a particularly high degree of scientific rigor as biases can easily be introduced that could affect the results. For example, someone who has been recently treated for cancer is more likely to remember stressful life events than someone without a cancer diagnosis, as the cancer patient is going to be searching for some reason to explain why he or she got the cancer. This is likely to bias any research finding.

One meta-analysis examined 165 different research studies of stress-related psychosocial factors and cancer incidence in initially healthy populations. It combined the results after excluding those studies that were not thought to be of adequate quality. Hundreds of thousands of subjects were included in the total and most studies followed these people for more than ten years.

The only cancer that was found to have an association with stress was lung cancer, and even here, the authors questioned the possibility of bias. There was no increased risk due to stress for breast, colon, stomach, lymphatic and blood, prostate, female genital, or skin cancers. The study, however, it did not exclude the possibility of a stress-prone personality or a poor coping style increasing cancer risk, and also depression could be a relevant factor

The Nurses' Health Study looked at work-related stress in 37,562 nurses and followed them for eight years. Over this time, 1,030 women were diagnosed with breast cancer. Their jobs were categorized into four levels from low stress to high stress. When analyzed, there was no difference in the rate of getting breast cancer with any of the job-stress categories. If anything, the higher stress jobs tended to be associated with less cancer risk. The study also analyzed for self-perceived job stress. Again, there were no differences in breast cancer rates for any of the perceived job-stress levels.

What You Should Do

- Stressful life events do not cause cancer. This is not a reason to change your job!
- There might be cancer-prone individuals, because of their stress-prone personality or lack of coping skills. Coping skills can be learned, so if appropriate, consider counseling services.

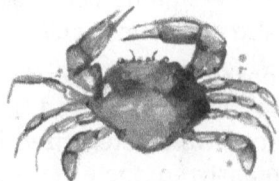

Vitamins and Minerals

Vitamins and minerals are essential for our cells to function properly. If they are in short supply, diseases can develop. For example, centuries ago, sailors often developed the disease scurvy after being at sea for months on end. Once it was found that scurvy was due to vitamin C deficiency and occurred because the sailors did not get fresh fruit, taking a supply of lemons and limes onboard solved the problem, as citrus is rich in vitamin C. There are many similar examples of vitamin deficiency and disease.

Perhaps originating from these situations, there is a general belief that taking vitamin and mineral supplements wards off disease. What is evident from research, however, is that the best way to ward off disease is to get your vitamins from what you eat, or in the case of vitamin D from the sun, rather than taking supplements.

This applies to cancer and other diseases, although there are some situations where taking extra vitamins in the form of supplements appears to help. In general, the dose of vitamins in a multivitamin preparation is considerably lower than when you buy an individual vitamin. Care must be taken with the use of vitamin supplements, as taking too much of some vitamins can cause disease or even cancer, as with vitamin A and lung cancer.

Vitamins

The Antioxidant Vitamins—A, C, and E

Vitamin A, its precursors beta-carotene and retinol, and vitamins C and E are all antioxidant vitamins. Antioxidants might reduce cancer risk, as they scavenge free oxide radicals that can damage DNA. They also stimulate immunity and promote cell differentiation, and these should also be protective.

Foods rich in antioxidants, especially fruits and vegetables, have been shown to reduce cancer risk in large population studies. These sort of observational studies, however, do not prove that the antioxidants are responsible for any reduction in cancer, as there are a lot of other potentially beneficial substances in fruits and vegetables. The best way to prove that something we take in is beneficial is a randomized trial of taking that substance compared to taking a placebo, continuing the study for years, then seeing if one group has a reduction in the rate of cancer.

Vitamin A, Carotenoids, and Retinol. Studies of vitamin A tend to include retinol and carotenoids, as these provitamins are metabolized to active vitamin A in the body. Vitamin A comes from animal and dairy food products, while beta-carotene sources include orange- and yellow-colored fruits and vegetables. Vitamin A and its provitamins are fat soluble, so they need fat in the diet to be absorbed. Once absorbed, they are stored in the liver, so we do not need to ingest these vitamins every day, as the liver will release them as needed.

Because they are not water soluble, any excess consumed cannot be easily dispensed through the kidneys. It is therefore possible for toxic levels to occur with vitamin A consumption. This does not apply to beta-carotene excess, as the body only converts it to vitamin A as needed. Excess beta-carotene can build up in the skin and cause yellowing, but it is not harmful. Excess vitamin A can do damage. It is important to avoid taking high-dose supplements of vitamin A, carotenoids, and retinoids.

Cohort studies have shown that having a high level of beta-carotene in the blood from dietary sources is associated with a lower risk of a number of cancers, possibly because of the antioxidant properties. However, when taken as a supplement, there is little evidence it can reduce cancer risk. Two RCTs of 50 mg of beta-carotene every second day for ten to twelve years did not show any reduction in cancer.

When beta-carotene was given to smokers, as researchers thought it might reduce their lung cancer risk, it did the opposite. In an RCT where smokers were given either a high dose of beta-carotene or a placebo, those who took the beta-carotene had a 20 percent increase in their risk of getting lung cancer. A similar increase in prostate cancer has been shown in another trial of beta-carotene. Once the beta-carotene was stopped, the risk increase diminished over time. This shows just how important it is to have proof of benefit before taking supplements.

There is some evidence that taking retinol might reduce skin cancer. One trial randomly allocated over 2,000 people with sun-damaged skin to take either 25,000 units of retinol by mouth daily or a placebo. Those taking retinol had a 25 percent reduction in the number of new skin squamous cancers they developed. However, those taking the retinol did have a rise in their triglyceride and cholesterol levels, so in theory, it might increase the risk of heart disease.

Vitamin C. There is no evidence that taking vitamin C supplements reduces cancer risk. Given that vitamin C is an antioxidant, this is a little surprising, but large randomized trials have not shown any reduction.

The Health Professionals Study, of nearly 15,000 males, and the Women's Antioxidant Cardiovascular Study, of over 7,500 women, randomized their participants to either 500 mg of vitamin C daily or a placebo. After eight to ten years, there was no cancer reduction in the vitamin C groups.

Vitamin E. Vitamin E is another antioxidant vitamin and, like vitamin C, there is no evidence that it plays any role in cancer prevention. The Women's Health Study randomized almost 40,000 healthy women to take either a placebo or vitamin E for ten years, and there was no increase or decrease in risk from any cancer. Other RCTs, including those in men, have not shown any cancer reduction benefit from vitamin E supplementation.

What You Should Do

- Have a diet containing plenty of fruits and vegetables, especially the yellow-orange type, as this will provide all your beta-carotene and other antioxidant vitamin needs.
- There is no proven cancer benefit in taking supplements of vitamins A, C, or E.
- Do not take high-dose vitamin A, beta-carotene, or retinol supplements, as they can be harmful.

The B Vitamins

There are a number of vitamins in the B group, including B1 (thiamine), B2 (riboflavin), B3 (nicotinamide or niacin), B6 (pyridoxine), and B12 (cyanocobalamin). Folic acid is also a B vitamin (sometimes called B9). They play an essential role in cell metabolism and can prevent some cancers.

The best source of B vitamins is meat, although cereals also contain some, but once cereals are refined, much of the B vitamin is lost. You might see flour labeled as "fortified" or "enriched," which means that B vitamins have been added to make up for that lost during processing. Legumes, such as beans, fruits, vegetables, nuts, and yeasts, are also sources of B vitamins. When taking B vitamin supplements, it is difficult to overdose, as the B vitamins are water soluble, so any excess is excreted in the urine.

Taking vitamin B supplements has been shown to reduce the chances of getting some cancers. In particular skin cancers, both malignant melanoma and the more common basal cell cancers and squamous cell cancers, have been shown to be prevented by regular B vitamin supplements. One meta-analysis of sixteen randomized trials of B vitamins, which involved 74,498 people, found that the rate of getting malignant melanoma was more than halved in those who took B vitamins. In this review, breast cancer was also reduced by nearly 20 percent, but there was no reduction in other cancers. This meta-analysis looked at B vitamin supplements in general and did not look at the individual B vitamins.

Vitamin B6

Vitamin B6 does appear to be important in cancer prevention. Dietary studies have shown that a high intake of vitamin B6 from foods is associated with a reduction in many cancers. In a meta-analysis, gastrointestinal cancers and particularly cancer of the esophagus, pancreas, stomach, and colon were reduced in those eating a diet rich in B6. Breast cancer was also reduced but not to the same extent. When researchers looked at blood levels of vitamin B6, people with high blood levels similarly had a reduction in these cancers, and also lung cancer was reduced. The higher the blood level of vitamin B6, the lower the cancer risk. Good food sources for vitamin B6 are bananas, nuts, and vegetables.

Vitamin B3

There has been a trial of vitamin B3 supplements that showed a reduction in the chances of getting nonmelanoma skin cancer. In this randomized trial of either vitamin B3 500 mg twice daily or a placebo, the people taking B3 had up to a 30 percent reduction in the chances of getting a new skin cancer. The group studied was 400 people who had already had a skin cancer and so were at higher risk. This dose of 500 mg twice daily is larger than in a B vitamin complex supplement, but it appears to be side-effect free.

Folate

Folate is one of the B-vitamin group and is important in DNA function and repair, so could well be important in cancer. It is found in green leafy vegetables, cereals, and nuts. Folic acid is the synthetic form of folate that is found in supplements.

A high dietary intake of folate has been shown to be associated with a decreased risk of a number of cancers, including cancers of the esophagus and pancreas, and both colorectal cancer and colonic polyps, a precursor of colon cancer. Studies have not, however, shown that taking folic acid supplements reduces cancer risk, and, as with vitamin A, it might even be harmful by increasing cancer risk. One RCT showed that the people randomized to take folic acid supplements had more advanced colorectal cancers than those taking a placebo, while others showed an increased risk of prostate cancer and an increase in the risk of death from cancer.

This information suggests that higher doses of folic acid supplementation might increase the rate at which a cancer grows. The dose of folic acid in these trials was in the range of 0.5–5 mg per day. This is much higher than the amount of folic acid we ingest from fortified flour or other cereals, which is most likely harmless from a cancer point of view and has definite noncancer health benefits.

What You Should Do

- Have a healthy diet, which includes whole grains, fruits, vegetables, and nuts, so that you have a good natural source of B vitamins.
- A daily supplement of B group vitamins might be beneficial in cancer prevention.
- If you have sun-damaged skin, vitamin B3 at a dose of 500 mg twice daily will help reduce skin cancer development and it appears to be harmless.
- Do not take folic acid supplements unless medically indicated, such as in pregnancy.

Vitamin D

We get most of our vitamin D from sunlight, not from our diet, as most foods contain only small amounts of vitamin D. Sunlight on our skin converts cholesterol to vitamin D3, but even this needs activation by enzymes in the liver to another form of vitamin D3 known as calcitriol. The best dietary sources of vitamin D3 are oily fish, liver, and egg yolks.

What vitamin D3 we do get from our diet is also converted to calcitriol in the liver. Calcitriol plays an important part in regulating cellular function, so it has the potential to affect cancer development. This includes cell growth, programmed cell death (apoptosis), blood vessel proliferation around cells, and inflammation. It also plays an important part in regulating bone metabolism and not enough can lead to osteoporosis.

Many people do not get enough sunlight UV exposure to maintain adequate vitamin D3 levels. Reasons include such things as them being concerned about the effect of sunlight exposure and skin cancer, populations who live near the North and South Poles naturally get less sunlight exposure, or some people have indoor occupations that do not allow much sun exposure. To get enough vitamin D3 through diet alone, you would need to eat large amounts of vitamin D3-rich foods daily. As not everyone gets enough sunlight on their skin to produce vitamin D3 or they do not eat enough vitamin D3-rich foods, it is common to take vitamin D3 as a dietary supplement to try to boost vitamin D3 levels.

The first indication that vitamin D3 might be important in cancer development came from the observation that people who lived in parts of the world far from the equator, and so had less sunlight exposure, were more likely to get colon and prostate cancers. This led to animal studies that showed that when cancer-prone mice were given vitamin D3 or calcitriol, the animals were less likely to get cancer. They also had reduced growth in any tumors that did develop.

Human studies have mostly studied circulating levels of vitamin D3 and subsequent cancer development. Colon cancer is 30–40 percent less likely to develop in people who have high blood levels of vitamin D3 compared to those with low levels. This is not so apparent with other types of cancer. However, someone who has already been treated for cancer, and who has higher circulating vitamin D3 levels, is less likely to have the cancer recur and die from the cancer than someone who has low levels. This has been reported for colon cancer, breast cancer, and prostate cancer.

From this, you would think that to raise vitamin D3 levels and protect yourself from cancer, you should take vitamin D3 as a supplement. In theory, yes. In practice, this is not so clear. There has only been one randomized trial where either vitamin D3 or a placebo has been given to a healthy population and the groups compared to see if the vitamin D3 group developed less cancer.

This was the VITAL study, where nearly 26,000 people were studied, with the vitamin D3 group taking 2,000 IU daily. They were followed for five years. The vitamin D3 group did not have any reduction in their incidence of cancer compared to the control group, but they did have a 25 percent reduction in the risk of dying from cancer.

This might be accounted for by the known biological action of vitamin D3 in reducing the aggressiveness of cancer cells and so the likelihood of metastasis. Why there was no reduction in cancer incidence is not known, but the five years of the study might not have been long enough to see any benefit from vitamin D3. For normal cells to become cancerous, then for those cells to form a visible or palpable tumor, is a process that normally takes more than five years.

How Much Sunlight Is Enough?

The amount of exposure to sunlight required to give you an adequate vitamin D3 level depends on a number of factors, including the following.

- **Sun intensity.** This is determined by whether it is summer or winter, and how far you live from the equator. There are a number of weather apps that can provide the UV level for the time of day, season, and your location.

- **Age.** Older people need more sun exposure, as their skin does not make vitamin D3 as well as the skin of young people.

- **Skin exposed.** How much is exposed and how long you are out in the sun. If you are using a UV-blocking cream, that will reduce your UV exposure.

- **Color of skin.** Dark-skinned people need more time in the sun to achieve an adequate vitamin D3 level, as do obese people.

In summer, about fifteen minutes of sun exposure on the face, arms, and hands each day might be enough if you are fair-skinned. In London, that would need to be about midday, while in Australia it should be earlier or later in the day to prevent burning. In winter, and if you are older or dark-skinned, longer sunlight exposure will be necessary to maintain adequate vitamin D3 levels. Note that glass blocks out UVB, so sitting in front of a window does not work!

What You Should Do

- Try to get some sun exposure on your skin every day. Sun exposure has been shown to prevent a number of diseases, not just cancer.
- If your vitamin D3 level is low despite getting sunlight, take 1,000 IU of vitamin D3 each day. This should only be the fallback option; maintaining vitamin D3 through sun exposure is better.
- If you have had cancer, and especially if you have had bowel cancer, maintaining your vitamin D3 level can help reduce the chances of the cancer returning. This should be a high priority, using whatever means you can, including sun exposure, diet, and supplementation.

Minerals

Calcium. Calcium is essential for cell function and has a wide variety of functions in the body, including bone structure, blood clotting, nerve transmission, and muscle contraction, including the heart muscle. Milk and cheese are the most important dietary sources, but almonds, greens, and sesame seeds also contain significant amounts.

Large cohort studies have shown that people who have a high calcium intake, in the order of more than 700 mg each day, have a 30–40 percent lower chance of getting colorectal cancer. This applies to intake from both dietary sources and supplements. In RCTs of calcium supplementation compared to a placebo, those taking calcium had a significantly lower chance of developing colonic polyps, which are a precursor to bowel cancer. On the downside, some studies have shown that calcium from dairy products might increase the risk of getting prostate cancer.

Selenium. Some decades ago, studies reported a lower risk of cancer in people who had a diet rich in selenium, or who had high levels in their blood. Follow-up laboratory studies showed that cancer cell growth was inhibited by selenium. More recent RCTs have, apart from the Linxian trial, failed to show that people taking selenium supplements had any reduction in their chances of getting cancer. The Linxian Nutrition Intervention Trial explored the possibility that in a region of China, which has a particularly high incidence of esophageal and stomach cancer and a low intake of several micronutrients, giving a combination of vitamin and trace element supplements might reduce this risk compared to a placebo.

Over 30,000 people were recruited and a variety of vitamin and trace element combinations were tested. The results showed that the combination of vitamin E, beta-carotene, and selenium did reduce cancer. Those taking this combination had a lower incidence of, and mortality from, esophageal and stomach cancers. There was a more than 10 percent reduction in cancer overall, and much of this was contributed to by a more than 20 percent reduction in stomach cancer. There was no benefit from other combinations that included retinol, zinc, B vitamins, vitamin C, and molybdenum.

Zinc. Zinc plays an important part in cell function and is important in cell reproduction and proliferation, and it also helps defend against free radicals. It is possible that zinc deficiency might weaken our defenses against cancer, and so it is not surprising that taking zinc supplements has been suggested as a way to ward off cancer.

Trials have not shown any cancer protection by taking zinc supplements, and some studies have shown that taking zinc might increase the risk of prostate cancer. The Health Professionals Follow-up Study of 47,000 men found that taking 100 mg of zinc daily resulted in more than a doubling of prostate cancer incidence. It was higher still in those who had taken the zinc for more than ten years. In the Linxian Nutrition Intervention study, a combination of retinol and zinc did not prevent esophageal or stomach cancers.

What You Should Do

- Maintain a high calcium intake through diet, supplements, or both, as this can help prevent colorectal cancer.
- Selenium supplements are probably only beneficial in areas of selenium deficiency, but in this situation, they can help reduce stomach and esophageal cancers.
- Taking zinc supplements has no cancer protection.

Vitamin and Mineral Supplements

Decrease or Increase Risk

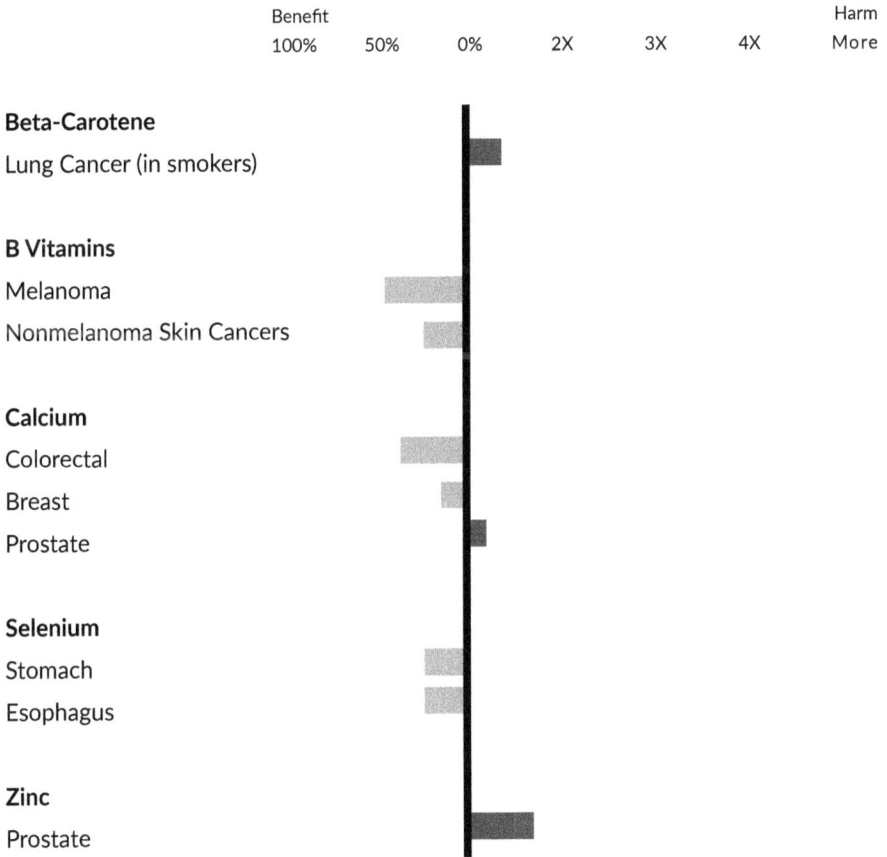

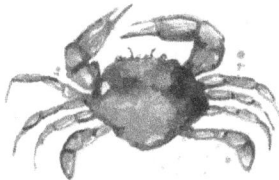

Benefit						Harm
100%	50%	0%	2X	3X	4X	More

Beta-Carotene

Lung Cancer (in smokers)

B Vitamins

Melanoma

Nonmelanoma Skin Cancers

Calcium

Colorectal

Breast

Prostate

Selenium

Stomach

Esophagus

Zinc

Prostate

Part 3—The Common Cancers

Gastrointestinal Tract Cancers

Liver Cancer

Pancreatic Cancer

The Female Cancers

The Male Cancers

Cancers of the Respiratory Tract

Cancers of the Urinary Tract

Skin Cancer

Thyroid Cancer

Brain Tumors

Blood and Lymphatic Cancers

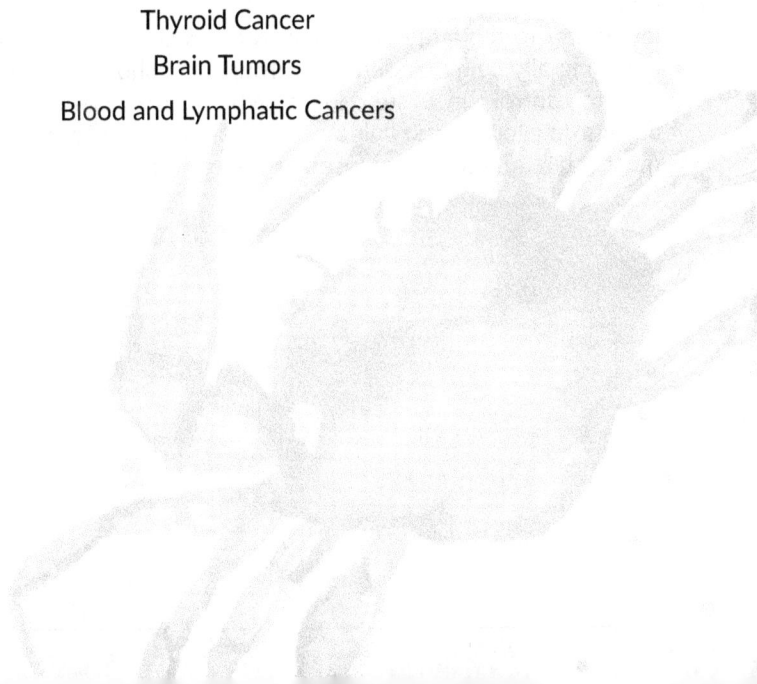

Gastrointestinal Tract Cancers

Cancer of the Oral Cavity

Esophageal Cancer

Gastric Cancer

Colorectal Cancer

Anal Cancer

The gut, or gastrointestinal tract as it is correctly known, is a long tube of muscle, lined by cells called epithelial cells, whose main function is to absorb digested food. It extends from the oral cavity, down the esophagus, which is a conduit to the stomach where the food is churned and partly digested. It is then slowly released into the small bowel, where most of the digestion and absorption takes place, then proceeds to the large bowel (or colon).

Here, there is a vast amount of bacterial activity that only recently has been recognized as an important part of body function. Eventually, it reaches the lower part of the large bowel called the rectum, where the residue is stored, before finally being passed out through the short anal canal, which acts as a gate to control the waste release. When cancer develops in the gut, it nearly always develops in the lining or epithelium, because it is this layer that is the most active and that is exposed to the contents.

Cancer of the Oral Cavity

What Is Oral Cavity Cancer?

The oral cavity has various components including the lips, cheeks, palate, gums, tongue, salivary glands, tonsils, and oropharynx. The oropharynx is the cavity at the back where food passes to the esophagus and inhaled air passes to the lungs after entering through the nasal passages or mouth.

The oral cavity is exposed to a whole range of carcinogens, being the first site of contact in the body of anything eaten or inhaled through the mouth. As a result, squamous cell cancers can develop. The squamous cell is the type of cell forming the surface lining, and it is this layer that gets exposed to inhaled or eaten carcinogens and undergoes malignant change.

Who Gets Oral Cavity Cancer?

Worldwide, there are about half a million cases each year, and it accounts for more than 3 percent of all cancers. They occur mostly in men and this most likely represents their higher rate of smoking. For the most part, the disease occurs as a result of a combination of smoking, alcohol consumption, and poor nutrition.

The regions with the highest incidence are Western Europe and South Central Asia, encompassing India, Bangladesh, Pakistan, and Sri Lanka, where over a quarter of all cases occur. In these Asian populations, chewing betel quid, sometimes with tobacco added, is a factor. In countries where smoking rates have decreased, there follows a fall in the rate of these cancers. In some affluent countries, however, there has been a rise due to increasing rates of oral HPV infection.

Preventing Oral Cavity Cancer

Smoking

Smoking is the major cause of cancer of the oral cavity. The longer a person smokes and the more frequently they smoke, the higher the risk. As with lung cancer, this is reversible. Someone who stopped smoking twenty years ago has a risk little different to a nonsmoker. Tobacco and betel quid chewing are also important causes of oral cavity cancer, especially in South Central Asia, while secondhand tobacco smoke is likely to also increase the risk.

Alcohol

Virtually every study that has looked at alcohol consumption and oral cavity cancer has confirmed that drinking alcohol increases the risk of getting oral cavity cancer, and this is especially so for heavy drinkers. Someone who drinks five to ten alcoholic drinks each day at least doubles their risk of getting this cancer.

Human Papillomavirus (HPV)

Oral HPV infection is an important cause of oral cavity cancer, especially in the oropharynx. It has been suggested that 70 percent of oropharyngeal cancers are due to oral HPV infections. The infection can be transmitted by mouth-to-genital or mouth-to-mouth contact. Vaccination for HPV, done to prevent cervical cancer, also helps prevent oral HPV infection and should prevent this cancer.

Diet

It is likely that a diet rich in vegetables, apart from starchy root vegetables, has a protective effect. One study showed a more than 30 percent reduction in risk for high consumers of these vegetables. For people who have a healthy diet overall, such as the Mediterranean diet, there is the same beneficial effect.

Coffee

People who drink three or more cups of coffee per day have a lower risk of oral cavity cancer, at least a 15 percent reduction.

Mate

Mate is a caffeine-rich drink prepared from an infusion of leaves using extremely hot water; it is drunk though much of South America. Studies have shown that people who drink a lot of mate have an increased risk of oral cavity cancer.

To Prevent Oral Cavity Cancer

- Do not smoke.
- Limit alcohol consumption.
- Eat fruits and vegetables.
- Drink three or more cups of coffee per day.
- Encourage childhood vaccination for HPV.

Esophageal Cancer

What Is Esophageal Cancer?

There are two main forms of cancer of the lining of the esophagus, and the type depends on where it occurs along this tube. Squamous cell cancer (SCC) tends to occur in the upper two-thirds, while adenocarcinoma is more common in the lower third. The most common form is SCC, but adenocarcinoma is becoming more common.

In both forms of the disease, something triggers the lining cells to grow in an uncontrolled manner so a mass of tissue is formed and eventually blocks the esophagus. Initially swallowing becomes difficult, then is no longer possible.

Esophageal cancer is the seventh most common cancer worldwide. It is estimated that there are over 600,000 cases annually. Unfortunately, few people survive this cancer. It is ranked the sixth most common cause of cancer death in the world.

Who Gets Esophageal Cancer?

About 80 percent of cases occur in less well-developed countries. Esophageal SCC is most common in a belt extending from Iran across the central Asian republics to China. It also occurs in Southern and Eastern Africa. In general, the rates of SCC of the esophagus have been declining worldwide, while adenocarcinoma has been increasing, particularly in Western countries.

Squamous Cell Carcinoma. It is thought that 90 percent of SCC of the esophagus is caused by a combination of smoking, alcohol, and a diet deficient in fruits and vegetables. In some parts of the world, vegetables are pickled and consumed in sufficient quantities that the N-nitroso compounds in the pickles damage DNA, predisposing the esophageal lining to become cancerous. Chewing of betel nuts with their leaves is common in Asia and is also believed to predispose to SCC of the esophagus.

On the other hand, a meta-analysis of multiple smaller studies has shown that eating fresh fruits and vegetables is protective. Drinking hot beverages, such as tea, particularly about 65 degrees C (150 degrees F) or more, is thought to cause burns to the esophagus. There are studies showing that this also increases the esophageal cancer risk.

Adenocarcinoma of the Esophagus. Acid reflux from the stomach into the lower esophagus is the main cause of adenocarcinoma. The body has mechanisms to prevent reflux, but these are not always effective. Acid reflux is more common in people who are overweight or obese, and the world's obesity epidemic accounts for much of the increasing incidence of adenocarcinoma.

This is probably just a simple pressure phenomenon where the mass of fat that has accumulated inside the abdomen puts pressure on the stomach, so gastric acid gets forced up the esophagus. It tends to be worse at night when lying flat—the help of gravity in keeping the acid in the stomach is removed and so it is more likely to move into the lower esophagus.

For most people, this is a nuisance and the discomfort can be relieved by taking an antacid or acid-suppressing medication. Occasionally, it is severe enough for the acid to reflux to the mouth and be inhaled while asleep, causing coughing or even lung damage.

In some people, acid reflux results in chronic inflammation of the lining of the lower esophagus. As a result, the squamous cells, which normally line the esophagus, change to be the stomach-type of columnar cells, a process called metaplasia. This change in the lining of the lower esophagus is visible at the time of an upper gastrointestinal endoscopy and is known as Barrett's esophagus.

The development of Barrett's esophagus is a risk factor for adenocarcinoma of the lower esophagus. The risk is generally assessed by taking biopsies of the Barrett's esophagus at the time of the endoscopy. The specimens are sent to the pathology laboratory where the pathologists will categorize it into Barrett's esophagus without dysplasia, with mild dysplasia (low grade), or with severe dysplasia (high grade).

Dysplasia is a measure of the cell damage as seen through the microscope. The more severe the dysplasia, the higher the cancer risk. It also depends on the extent of the changes, with long segments of change being at higher risk. It is estimated that someone who has Barrett's esophagus has a 2 in 1,000 chance of developing adenocarcinoma of the esophagus each year. For someone with mild dysplasia on biopsy, this rises to over 5 per 1,000 per year, and for severe dysplasia it is as high as 40 to 80 per 1,000 cases each year!

Preventing Esophageal Cancer

Preventing Squamous Cell Carcinoma

Squamous carcinoma of the esophagus is common in parts of the world where smoking, alcohol consumption, and a diet low in fruits and vegetables are part of the culture. Prevention requires public health education programs to educate about the dangers of this combination of factors and encourage change.

Smoking

Smoking is a significant factor, with current smokers having a 50 percent increased risk of developing esophageal cancer. Stopping smoking reduces this risk.

Alcohol

Alcohol, particularly spirits but also beer, plays a significant role in causing squamous cancer of the esophagus. For every 10 gm consumed each day, the risk rises by 25 percent. Regular drinkers double their risk, while one meta-analysis showed that people who drank seven alcoholic drinks per day had their risk increased tenfold. The combination of smoking and alcohol is worse than one alone.

Diet

Eat fruits and vegetables. People who consume a diet rich in fruits and vegetables, particularly green vegetables, have a 10-20 percent lower risk of getting squamous cancer compared to those who consume little.

HPV Vaccination

The human papillomavirus (HPV) is known to cause most cases of cervical cancer; it is also a cause of oral and anal cancers. It can also cause squamous cancer of the esophagus. It should be preventable by vaccination, and HPV vaccines are now widely available.

Preventing Adenocarcinoma of the Esophagus

Treat Reflux

Adenocarcinoma is becoming more common in affluent societies, most likely due to the rising rates of overweight and obesity. It can be effectively prevented by controlling acid reflux into the lower esophagus. One problem, however, is that not everyone who has reflux knows they have it. It can occur without any symptoms.

Once diagnosed, reflux should be treated, particularly if Barrett's esophagus is present. Aggressive antireflux treatments have been shown to decrease the chances of adenocarcinoma of the esophagus from developing.

Treatment usually includes medication, such as a proton pump inhibitor (PPI) that reduces acid production, and this needs to be continued long term. Weight loss should also help. In patients who prove to be resistant to a PPI and continue to have reflux, antireflux surgery should be considered and this is usually done by keyhole, minimally invasive surgery.

Aspirin

Aspirin is useful in the prevention of a number of cancers and has been shown to reduce the development of Barrett's esophagus in people with reflux. It also reduces the occurrence of esophageal cancer in people with Barrett's esophagus.

Treat Barrett's Esophagus

Once Barrett's esophagus has been diagnosed, apart from being treated aggressively, it should be monitored by regular endoscopy. How often this should occur depends on the severity of any dysplasia. The aim is to detect cancer at an early stage, should it occur.

If there is no dysplasia, an endoscopy every three years should suffice. With low-grade dysplasia, it should be treated with intense PPI therapy for a few months, then have a repeat endoscopy and biopsies. With persisting or high-grade dysplasia, endoscopic treatment by radiofrequency ablation should be undertaken. Regular post-treatment endoscopy should continue, to detect incomplete treatment or recurrence of the Barrett's esophagus.

To Prevent Squamous Esophageal Cancer

- Don't smoke.
- Limit alcohol consumption.
- Eat fruits and vegetables.
- Encourage childhood vaccination for HPV.

To Prevent Adenocarcinoma Esophageal Cancer

- Treat gastroesophageal reflux.
- Lose excess body fat.
- Treat Barrett's esophagus.

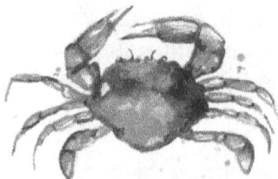

Gastric Cancer

What Is Gastric Cancer?

Gastric cancer, also known as stomach cancer, occurs when the cells lining the stomach undergo malignant change and grow in an uncontrolled fashion. To begin with, this growth is just into the stomach wall, but later cells spread through the lymph channels and blood vessels to other parts of the body. Unfortunately, all too often, it has no symptoms until spread has occurred, making cure rarely possible.

There are a number of variants of gastric cancer, although their behavior is not a lot different. The most common form occurs in the lower stomach as an ulcer and is particularly common in China and Japan. This sort is referred to as noncardia gastric cancer and it is becoming less common.

The next type occurs in the upper stomach near where the esophagus enters and is similar to adenocarcinoma of the esophagus described in the previous section. It is called gastric cardia cancer. It is becoming more common and is the variety most seen in Western countries.

A third variety does not form a lump or ulcer but grows diffusely through the stomach wall over a large area and is called linitis plastica. Fortunately, it is uncommon, and it is rarely survived, as it is usually diagnosed late.

Gastric cancer is the fifth most common cancer, and worldwide there are about a million cases per year. It is the third most common cause of cancer death. There are a number of mechanisms for its causation, with several factors making the stomach lining more susceptible to cancer. Chronic *Helicobacter pylori* infection can result in the stomach lining producing less acid, as can high-salt foods. This reduced acid production results in less vitamin C absorption. Gastrin, a stomach hormone, production is also stimulated, and this can result in proliferation of cells.

Another effect of reduced acid production is that it allows the growth of undesirable bacteria that can convert nitrites in preserved foods into carcinogenic N-nitroso compounds. Chronic inflammation also predisposes the stomach lining to cancerous change.

Who Gets Gastric Cancer?

Noncardia Gastric Cancer

Noncardia gastric cancer occurs most commonly in East Asia and about 50 percent of the world's cases occur in China. It occurs predominantly in men who smoke and drink, and in particular, it is the consumption of preserved foods that is believed to play an important role in its causation.

The main reason these cancers are becoming less common is the more widespread use of refrigeration for food storage, rather than pickling or preservation with salt. People who have long-term stomach infections with *Helicobacter pylori* are another group who are prone to noncardia cancer.

Cardia Gastric Cancer

Cancer of the gastric cardia, in the upper part of the stomach, is more common in Western societies. Unlike noncardia gastric cancer, it is becoming more common and it is just as lethal as noncardia gastric cancer. Like adenocarcinoma of the esophagus, it relates to obesity and acid reflux, although it is not necessarily associated with Barrett's esophagus.

Preventing Gastric Cancer

Alcohol

Regular consumption of alcohol, particularly three or more drinks per day (45 gm of alcohol), increases the risk of stomach cancer, and the risk increases steadily for every subsequent drink. Alcohol is broken down into acetaldehyde and this is known to be a carcinogen, having a direct effect on the lining of the stomach.

Diet: Fruit Consumption

A low intake of fruit, citrus fruit in particular, is associated with an increased stomach cancer risk. For example, someone who eats no fruit has a 20 percent higher risk than someone who eats two portions per day. For citrus, the benefit is a 25 percent lower cancer risk for each 100 gm eaten, although this is mainly for cancer of the gastric cardia. Fruit, particularly citrus, contains vitamin C and many other antioxidants that help protect the stomach from cancer.

Diet: Preserved Foods

Salt-preserved vegetables are commonly eaten in Asia, where traditionally brine or soy sauce is used for the pickling. Compared to those who do not eat much, those with a large consumption of salt-preserved vegetables have a 30 percent increase in risk of getting stomach cancer. Processed meat consumption, such as bacon, salami, and ham, also results in an increase in stomach cancer risk.

Much the same applies for salt-preserved fish consumption, although the risk with fish is lower. The effect of salt in the diet seems to work together with *Helicobacter pylori* infection to cause chronic inflammation of the stomach lining, and so increase cancer risk. Many of these foods, particularly processed meats, also have high levels of nitrates and nitrites. In the stomach, these can change to become carcinogenic N-nitroso compounds.

Smoking

Smokers are at significantly increased risk of getting stomach cancer. A large meta-analysis showed that smokers, particularly male smokers, had a more than 50 percent increased chance of developing the disease. This risk has been shown to decrease ten years after cessation.

Helicobacter Pylori

Helicobacter pylori is a bacterium that lives in the stomach. It is common, found in about 35 percent of people in Western countries, while in parts of Asia it is present in as much as 90 percent of the population. Most people with this infection do not know they have it, although in some people it causes stomach ulcers, which can be painful.

It was only identified as a cause of disease in 1982 by Barry Marshall and Robin Warren who found it was linked to gastritis and gastric ulcers. Subsequent research has found that *Helicobacter pylori* might be linked to a whole range of diseases, both in the intestine and elsewhere in the body. These Australian scientists faced skepticism about their claim that *Helicobacter pylori* caused stomach ulcers, and eventually proved it by Marshall drinking a vial of cultured organisms. He became unwell and a gastroscopy showed stomach ulcers with *Helicobacter pylori* in his stomach. They were awarded the Nobel Prize in Physiology or Medicine for their discovery in 2005.

It is estimated that 1-2 percent of people who have long-term *Helicobacter pylori* infections will develop noncardia stomach cancer, and the longer they have it, the greater the risk. Damage to the stomach lining by *Helicobacter pylori* can manifest as inflammation or eventually atrophy, a situation where the lining cells reduce in number, flatten, and become nonfunctional, so the stomach no longer produces acid. This process is known as atrophic gastritis.

People with these changes plus *Helicobacter pylori* infection are at even higher risk of developing gastric cancer, with about one in three developing the disease. The combination of atrophic gastritis and *Helicobacter pylori* infection can be identified by a screening test. It is a combination of measuring blood levels of pepsinogen, a hormone that is low in people with extensive atrophic gastritis, and testing for *Helicobacter pylori* by either breath or stool testing.

Early eradication of *Helicobacter pylori* infection reduces the cancer risk. There has been a global decline in *Helicobacter pylori* infections and this might, in part, account for the global decline in noncardia stomach cancer.

Treatment is a relatively simple matter of taking a one-week course of a mixture of antibiotics, although antibiotic resistant *Helicobacter pylori* is now appearing. Yogurt-type bacteria, Lactobacillus and Bifidobacteria, improve the eradication rate as they tend to suppress *Helicobacter pylori*.

Excess Body Fat

People who are overweight have an increased chance of developing gastric cardia cancer, but there is no increased risk for the development of noncardia cancer. Excess body fat is usually measured by BMI (body mass index), with a BMI above 25 being regarded as overweight and a BMI over 30 being regarded as obese. For every five points of BMI above the normal upper limit of 25, the risk of cardia gastric cancer rises by about 25 percent.

To Prevent Gastric Cancer

- Don't smoke.
- Limit alcohol consumption.
- Eat fruit.
- Limit consumption of preserved foods.
- Lose excess fat.
- Treat *Helicobacter pylori* infection.

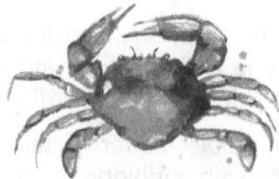

Colorectal Cancer

What Is Colorectal Cancer?

The colon and rectum together form the large bowel and while they might have different names, basically they are part of the same organ. The rectum is just the lower end where the stool is stored before evacuation. Digested food is mostly liquid when it enters the top end of the large bowel, the cecum, and as the muscles of the bowel wall slowly move this food residue toward the rectum, fluid is absorbed so the content becomes thicker.

The colon contains vast quantities of organisms known as the microbiome. For the most part, they are good bacteria, and these are increasingly being recognized as playing an important part in maintaining the body's health. Cancer in the colon and rectum are a little different in their behavior, but this is minimal, and they will be dealt with together.

Because the large bowel lining is in intimate contact with what food residue is passing through, it is logical that carcinogens in the food could result in the cells changing to become malignant. While this is important, there are many other factors that can influence colorectal cancer development. Once the cancer has formed, it grows within the bowel wall and in time might obstruct the bowel. Eventually, cells break off and move through either the lymphatic system to the lymph nodes along the blood vessels, or through the blood to more distant parts of the body. In particular, the liver is a common site of spread.

Who Gets Colorectal Cancer?

Worldwide, there are 1.8 million cases of colorectal cancer each year. It is the second most common cancer in women and the third most common in men. It is a disease of developed countries, where about one in twenty-four people will get colorectal cancer at some stage in their lives, and more so in men. The incidence in Western countries is about ten times that of West African countries. As poorer countries develop and become more Westernized in their lifestyles, colorectal cancer becomes more common. It has been estimated there will be a 60 percent increase worldwide over the next fifteen years.

Lifestyle, particularly diet, plays an important part in determining who gets colorectal cancer. People who eat a diet containing processed meats and red meat, and those who have more than two alcoholic drinks per day, are more susceptible. Eating a diet containing whole grains, fiber, and dairy products tends to protect the bowel from cancer. Apart from what we eat, low levels of physical activity, excess body fat, and smoking all increase colorectal cancer risk.

Another important factor for some people, and something you cannot do much about, is your genes. Some people inherit a genetic mutation that makes them more susceptible to bowel cancer. About 5 percent of large bowel cancers are thought to occur as a result of an inherited genetic mutation. For the most part, these occur as part of what we call a familial syndrome, that is, where a disease pattern occurs in a family.

One of these is familial adenomatous polyposis (FAP), where family members get large numbers of adenomatous polyps in their large bowel. Not all bowel polyps are adenomatous. A pathologist looking into a microscope can tell what sort it is, but adenomatous polyps are an early precursor of colorectal cancer. Before long, some of these polyps become malignant. This usually occurs before forty years of age, the result being colorectal cancer.

The other main inherited syndrome is hereditary nonpolyposis colorectal cancer (HNPCC), also known as Lynch syndrome. In this syndrome, there is a high incidence of colorectal cancer, often at a relatively young age, but without the prodromal polyp formation. These people are also more prone to cancers at other body sites.

One of the most important risk factors for getting colorectal cancer is again something we cannot do anything about, getting older. Colorectal cancer becomes more common with each succeeding decade. In recent years, there has been a trend toward this cancer becoming more common in young adults, sometimes appearing in the twenties or thirties. In the US, this increase has been at the rate of 2 percent for each year since 1990. The reason for this is not certain but might well be because of increasing obesity.

Another group of people who are at high risk of developing colorectal cancer are those people who have chronic inflammatory bowel disease (IBD). IBD is the group name for ulcerative colitis and Crohn's disease, conditions of uncertain cause where the bowel becomes chronically inflamed. Malignant change is more common in those people who have the whole large bowel inflamed and who have had the disease for many years. Those with active IBD for twenty years or more will develop large bowel cancer at a rate of 1 percent per year.

Preventing Colorectal Cancer

Treatment of colorectal cancer involves major surgery, sometimes with a stoma—the bowel being brought to the surface so it empties into a bag, and often requires chemotherapy. Despite treatment, it still has a high mortality. In the US, only about 60 percent of treated patients survive five years. It is worth preventing!

Diet

Given there is direct contact between what we eat and our gut wall, it is logical to think that the type of foods we put into our gut might in some way influence cancer development. Numerous studies have investigated this, with the aim that if we can find what it is in our diet that might cause cancer, then removing it will prevent the disease.

The World Cancer Research Fund has put together many of the best scientists in the world to analyze the information from all these studies, not only for bowel cancer but for a whole range of other cancers, and many of the recommendations provided here come from their reports.

Whole Grains. Virtually all studies of whole-grain consumption come to the same conclusion: that eating whole grains reduces colorectal cancer risk. Eating 90 gm of whole grains each day diminishes the risk by nearly 20 percent. Whole grains are an important source of bioactive compounds and vitamins that could have a protective effect. Whole grains are also an important source of fiber that not only increases the rate of transit through the gut, so there is less time for the contents to be in contact with the bowel wall, but also fiber is an important source of food for the intestinal bacteria that might in turn protect the bowel.

It is likely that much of the benefit comes from the bran and germ components of whole grains, and these are mostly removed during processing into flour. In a study where participants were randomly assigned to supplement their diet with unprocessed wheat bran or not, the bran group developed significantly fewer polyps than the control group, with colonic polyps being a precursor of colorectal cancer.

Fruits and Vegetables. Nearly all studies have shown that eating fruits and vegetables helps protect against colorectal cancer. Beneficial vegetables are not the starchy root vegetables, such as potato and sweet potato, but leafy and flowering types, also legumes. People who eat little or no vegetable matter have a 10-15 percent higher risk of getting colorectal cancer than those who eat 200-300 gm each day. Eating more than this only conveys a small additional benefit.

Red and Processed Meat. A high consumption of both red meat and preserved meats is associated with an increased risk of colorectal cancer. Nearly every study has shown this detrimental effect. Red meat is generally cooked at high temperatures and this can result in the formation of heterocyclic amines and polycyclic aromatic hydrocarbons, both of which have been shown to cause cancer in animal studies. Processed meats are mostly derived from red meat and might contain chemicals used as preservatives or absorbed in the smoking process. They can also contain N-nitroso compounds, know to promote cancer formation.

For red meat, the risk of getting colorectal cancer increases by up to 20 percent for each 100 gm of red meat eaten on average each day. This is more so in men than women, and the effect is more so on the colon, rather than the rectum. For preserved meats, for every 50 gm eaten on average per day, the risk increases by 20 percent, and this applies to women and men.

Fish. Fish consumption reduces colorectal cancer risk. People who eat on average 100 gm of fish per day have a 10 percent reduction in risk. Fish contains long chain omega-3 polyunsaturated fatty acids that have an anti-inflammatory action, so it could reduce cancer risk by that mechanism.

Dairy and Calcium. Nearly all studies have shown that people who consume dairy products have a lower risk of developing colorectal cancer. The risk progressively diminishes for every 100 gm consumed each day, until when consuming 500 gm per day, the risk is reduced by 20 percent compared to someone who has little dairy consumption. It is possible that it is the calcium in dairy that provides the benefit.

Dietary calcium is known to have a number of functions that inhibit bowel cancer formation. For a start, calcium binds to the bile acids and free fatty acids produced during the digestive process, preventing their toxicity on the bowel wall. It also promotes cell differentiation, something that has the opposite effect to cancer formation.

While calcium from food appears to protect against bowel cancer, does taking calcium supplements do the same thing? Overall the evidence is yes, there is a worthwhile benefit, although in the Women's Health Initiative study where women were randomly allocated to 1,000 mg calcium each day or a placebo over a period of seven years, there was no benefit.

Vitamins. Vitamin D is potentially beneficial in preventing a number of different cancers, as it important in controlling cell growth, reducing inflammation, and it improves immune function. Studies have shown that both vitamin D-containing foods and taking vitamin D supplements reduces the risk of developing colorectal cancer. Further research has also shown that people with higher levels of vitamin D in their blood have a lower risk.

Vitamin B6 (pyridoxine) has been shown in studies of both consumption and blood levels to be protective for colorectal cancer. Folic acid is another vitamin that has been linked to colorectal cancer. While some studies have shown that taking folate supplements reduced the number of colonic polyps and cancers, other studies showed an increase in colorectal cancer in people taking it, so folate supplementation should be avoided.

Proinflammatory Diet. One study took a novel way of approaching the issue of diet and colorectal cancer. The researchers developed an empirical dietary inflammatory pattern (EDIP) score and used the Nurses' Health Study and the Health Professionals Follow-up Study as their sources of data. They investigated if a proinflammatory diet, years earlier, could affect the number of colorectal cancers that subsequently developed.

We know that chronic inflammation can cause a variety of cancers, and the researchers developed their EDIP score by comparing dietary patterns in eighteen different food groups to three know inflammatory markers that can be measured in the blood: IL-6, CRP and TNFR2. Lower EDIP scores indicated a diet that is anti-inflammatory, while higher scores indicated a proinflammatory diet.

Processed meat, red meat, meat from organs, fish, refined grains, starchy vegetables, high-energy drinks, and tomatoes were associated with a high EDIP score (proinflammatory). Beer, wine, tea, coffee, yellow and green vegetables, and fruit juice were associated with a lower anti-inflammatory score. Compared to people eating the more anti-inflammatory diets, those with the highest proinflammatory diets had a 44 percent higher chance of developing colorectal cancer if male, and a 22 percent higher chance if female.

To minimize the chances of getting colorectal cancer by dietary means.

- Eat at least 90 gm of whole grains per day. If whole grains are too difficult, then a coarse muesli is a convenient way to get whole grains. Alternatively, supplement with wheat germ and unprocessed bran.
- Restrict the number of times you eat red meat and processed meats. Make up for this loss of protein source by eating fish.
- Eat at least 250 gm of fresh fruits and non-starchy vegetables each day.
- Consume dairy products, at least 200–300 gm per day. If that is not possible then supplement with calcium.
- Get adequate sunlight. Vitamin D appears to help, so eat vitamin D-rich foods such as fatty types of fish, liver, and egg yolks. If these do not give adequate vitamin D levels, take vitamin D supplements.
- Take vitamin B6 supplements.

Alcohol

Alcohol consumption increases colorectal cancer risk. At low levels of consumption, one standard drink per day, the risk is small. At two standard drinks per day (30 gm of alcohol), there is a 15 percent increase in risk. The higher the alcohol intake, the higher the risk. It does not seem to matter if it is wine, beer, or spirits. To reduce bowel cancer risk, alcohol consumption should be limited.

Physical Activity

Physically active people have up to a 20 percent lower risk of developing bowel cancer compared to those who are least active, although this applies mainly to colon cancer and not rectal cancer. This holds for both recreational physical activity and total daily physical activity. It is difficult to give a level of recreational activity needed for benefit, but a minimum is ten MET hrs/week, or thirty minutes of moderate activity, five days a week.

In reality, this level of activity will only slightly reduce risk. Achieving a greater benefit requires more dedication to an exercise program. One theory as to why colon, breast, and other cancers, in addition to heart disease and diabetes, have become so common in Western populations is that several hundred years ago most of the population had physically active jobs. We have now moved to a sedentary lifestyle.

Excess Body Fat

There have been at least 57 research studies of BMI and colorectal cancer, and nearly all have shown a positive link. Someone with a BMI of 30 has a 34 percent greater risk of developing colorectal cancer. Excess body fat seems more important in the development of colon cancer than rectal cancer, but it is still important for both. Other ways of measuring excess body fat, such as waist circumference or waist-hip ratio, show these also are markers of colorectal cancer risk increase.

A possible mechanism relates to insulin and its effect on growth factors, in particular IGF-1, which can stimulate the growth of colon cancer cells. Higher body fat levels are associated with increased insulin. Diabetics have a higher rate of developing colorectal cancer; a 40 percent higher risk for colon cancer and a 20 percent increased risk for rectal cancer.

Aspirin

Long-term use of low-dose aspirin, 100 mg each day, lowers the risk of developing colonic polyps and colorectal cancer, and it lowers the risk of dying after colorectal cancer has been treated. Multiple randomized trials have shown that taking aspirin for at least ten years reduces colorectal cancer risk by 20–40 percent, depending on the trial. People with Lynch syndrome, who are at a particularly high risk, have an even greater benefit with about a 50 percent reduction.

Smoking

Cigarette smokers have just under a 20 percent increased chance of getting both colorectal cancers and polyps.

Treat Precancerous Lesions

Remove colonic polyps. Adenomatous polyps are common precancerous lesions found growing on the wall of the large bowel. In the US, they are found in 20–30 percent of middle-aged people, and they become even more common with advancing age. Most people who have them are not aware they have them, as they rarely cause any symptoms. Not all polyps are the adenomatous variety, metaplastic and inflammatory polyps are harmless.

These outgrowths from the bowel wall might develop into cancers. It has been estimated that this will happen in about one in twenty adenomatous polyps. Understandably, this is difficult to determine because when a polyp is found, it is removed. Sometimes when a polyp is removed and sent to the laboratory for analysis, a small cancer is found to have already started. We get some idea which polyps are more at risk of changing, as they tend to be larger than a centimeter and have microscopic changes of high-grade dysplasia or a villous polyp change, a frond-like appearance as seen through a microscope.

Polyps start for much the same reasons as colorectal cancer and can be regarded as its first stages, although they are not yet malignant so they do not have the ability to spread through the body like a cancer. Not all adenomatous polyps go on to become cancers. When they do, it is often many years before this happens, so if removed, the chance of developing cancer is greatly reduced.

This is the basis for regular colonic screening. One study of nearly 1,500 people who had one or more polyps found on a routine colonoscopy, showed that those who had their polyps removed had a 90 percent lower chance of subsequently developing colorectal cancer in the next six years compared to those who did not.

This is a big reduction in cancer risk and so routine colonoscopy should be seriously considered for high-risk populations, particularly Western countries for people age fifty and older. It is normally recommended every five to ten years but should be more often if at higher risk, such as multiple previous polyps, a family history of colorectal cancer, or if previously treated for colorectal cancer.

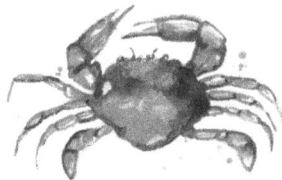

To Prevent Colorectal Cancer

- Your diet should include these foods.
  Whole grains, 90 gm per day.
  Limited red and processed meats. Eat fish instead.
  Fresh fruits and non-starchy vegetables, 300 gm per day.
  Dairy products, 250 gm per day, or calcium supplements.
  Vitamin D-rich foods or vitamin D supplements.
  Vitamin B6-rich foods or B6 supplements.
- Limit alcohol consumption.
- Be physically active, a minimum of ten MET/hours/week.
- Take low-dose aspirin daily, unless bleeding risk.
- Do not smoke.
- Have any colonic polyps removed at regular colonoscopy screenings.

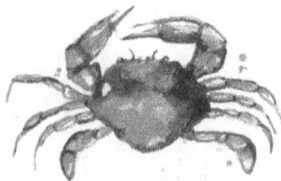

Anal Cancer

What Is Anal Cancer?

Anal cancer is not a common disease but the reason it is included in this book is that it is easily prevented. Nearly all cancers of the anal canal are squamous cell cancers, arising in the modified skin of the lower anal canal. They become apparent as a lump, pain, or bleeding. While years ago, treatment was by major surgery, the modern treatment is by chemotherapy and radiation therapy without surgery, and this often results in a cure. While rare, in the US, the incidence has doubled in a period of twenty years.

Who Gets Anal Cancer?

It is more common in men who have sex with men, in human immunodeficiency (HIV)-positive people, people with multiple sexual partners, and in those who have had genital warts or other sexually transmitted diseases. In women, there is a strong relationship to cervical cancer. All these factors are indicators of a higher risk of HPV infection.

More than 90 percent of anal squamous cell cancers are associated with an HPV virus infection. It is often HPV 16, the same virus subtype that also causes cervical cancer.

Preventing Anal Cancer

Vaccines that target the types of HPV infection associated with cervical and anal cancer have been developed. Preliminary studies indicate there is significant regression of precancerous lesions in men after vaccination. An HPV vaccine is available, and in many parts of the world, this is being offered to children, with two injections at least six months apart. In time, if near-universal vaccination can be achieved, anal cancer should be largely eliminated.

To Prevent Anal Cancer

- Encourage HPV vaccination.
- Practice safe sex.

Liver Cancer

What Is Liver Cancer?

Liver cancer, also known as hepatocellular cancer, occurs when the cells of the liver, the hepatocytes, undergo malignant change. Instead of doing their normal job of detoxifying the blood, they grow in an uncontrolled manner. This is primary cancer of the liver and not to be confused with secondary liver cancer, which starts somewhere else and spreads by the blood to seed and grow in the liver.

Who Gets Liver Cancer?

Hepatocellular cancer is a major source of disease and death worldwide and it is the fifth most common cancer in men and the ninth in women. It is the second-leading cause of cancer death in the world. As many as one million people get the disease each year—and die from it—as it has almost 100 percent mortality. About 80 percent of all cases have a common origin—chronic infections with the hepatitis B or hepatitis C viruses, so there is enormous potential for prevention.

About two billion people worldwide have had a hepatitis B infection, although most clear the infection spontaneously. It is spread by blood contact, often at birth, and it is most common in East Asia and Africa. In some people, the infection persists and becomes chronic, and these people have a hundredfold increase in their chances of getting hepatocellular cancer compared to noncarriers of the virus. There is a vaccine for the hepatitis B virus, and vaccination can markedly reduce the chances of becoming infected with the virus.

Hepatitis C infections are more common in high-income countries. The virus is spread by blood. It is more likely to become chronic compared to hepatitis B. In people with chronic hepatitis C infections, up to 4 percent will develop liver cancer each year. While there are no vaccines to prevent hepatitis C, there are effective antiviral drugs that can rid the body of the virus.

There are a number of other things that have been shown to increase the risk of getting liver cancer, so avoiding these can also reduce the risk. These only account for a small number of cases, compared to chronic hepatitis infections. They include aflatoxins, cirrhosis of the liver, long-term use of oral contraceptive with high-dose estrogen and progestin, alcohol intake, and excess body fat. On the other hand, people who consume three or more cups of coffee each day halve their chances of getting liver cancer.

Preventing Liver Cancer

Preventing hepatitis B by vaccination and receiving early active treatment of hepatitis C infections are the best way to prevent hepatocellular cancer.

Hepatitis B

Of the two billion people in the world who have been exposed to the hepatitis B virus, it is estimated that about 250 million are chronic carriers of the virus. It is these people who are at risk of developing hepatocellular cancer. The chance of developing liver cancer depends on the amount of active virus in the body, with those people who have high levels of active virus at the greatest risk.

The frequency of chronic hepatitis B varies from region to region in the world. In the US and most Western countries, the rate is less than 2 percent. In Asia and parts of South America, it is 2–7 percent. In Western Africa and South Sudan, more than 8 percent of the population have chronic hepatitis B infection.

The hepatitis virus can be transmitted from someone who is a carrier to someone who has no immunity. Vaccination provides the immunity to prevent this transmission. For most of the world, and especially areas where the disease is common, the hepatitis B virus is most commonly spread from a chronically infected mother to her child, and the transmission can occur before or during birth. This will occur in 90 percent of situations where there has been no immunization.

If the newborn is given hepatitis B immunoglobulin and is vaccinated within twelve hours of delivery, the chances of the child becoming infected is reduced by 95 percent. The risk is highest for women with a high viral load and in this situation, giving the pregnant mother antiviral therapy further reduces the risk of transmission to the infant. Many countries now have programs in place to do this. As a result, the rate of chronic hepatitis B infection, and subsequent liver cancer, is expected to dramatically reduce. The virus is not transmitted by breastfeeding.

In Western countries where hepatitis B is less common, the most common mode of transmission of the virus is by unprotected sexual contact or shared needles in IV drug users. For these high-risk groups or any workers who come into contact with body fluids, such as the healthcare profession, vaccination is actively encouraged.

Unlike hepatitis C, there are no known drugs that can cure hepatitis B. However, researchers are reportedly close to developing drugs that will do this.

Hepatitis C

Hepatitis C is less common than hepatitis B but is still an important cause of hepatocellular cancer. Worldwide, it is estimated that about 71 million people have chronic hepatitis C infection. Up to a quarter of people with chronic hepatitis C infections will go on to develop liver cancer and eventually die as a result. Liver cancer is even more common in people with both hepatitis B and hepatitis C infections, with 40 percent of such cases developing liver cancer in due course.

Successful treatment of hepatitis C is associated with a lower chance of developing hepatocellular cancer, although the risk is not completely eliminated. Since 2016, there have been new antiviral drugs available that target the hepatitis C virus. These are highly effective and do not have many of the unpleasant side effects compared to previous drugs. More than 95 percent of people treated are free of the virus after eight to twelve weeks of drug treatment.

The World Health Organization recommends that all people over twelve who have chronic hepatitis C infection be treated with a combination of direct-acting antiviral drugs that can kill all six major subtypes of the hepatitis C virus. Production costs of these drugs are low. There are currently no vaccines to prevent hepatitis C.

Toxins

Cirrhosis of the liver results from long-term liver cell damage. The liver becomes shrunken and nodular and does not function properly. Causes not only include chronic hepatitis B and C infections, but also toxic substances. Some toxins increase cancer risk without cirrhosis. Each year, one in every hundred people who have cirrhosis of the liver will develop hepatocellular cancer.

Alcohol is the most common toxin to cause liver cirrhosis. Another is aflatoxin, which can be a contaminant in stored corn, peanuts, and soybeans but, in reality, it is only responsible for a tiny fraction of liver cancers. It needs to be ingested in large amounts to be dangerous. Obesity, and its associated nonalcoholic fatty liver disease, is also associated with an increased risk of liver cancer. Iron can be toxic too, if it accumulates in the liver in large amounts as might occur in the hereditary disease of haemochromatosis. Avoiding these toxins reduces the risk of developing hepatocellular cancer.

Coffee

People who drink three or more cups of coffee per day reduce their chances of getting liver cancer by almost half. This applies to people who have chronic liver disease and those who do not, and it has been confirmed in numerous studies. What is not clear is how much is due to the caffeine, and how much is due to the large amount of antioxidants in coffee. Some studies suggest the benefit is from both caffeinated and decaffeinated coffees, while others indicate it might just be with caffeinated coffee.

To Prevent Liver Cancer

- Vaccinate for hepatitis B, if at risk.
- Treat hepatitis C, if infected.
- Avoid toxin excess, such as alcohol.
- Drink coffee.

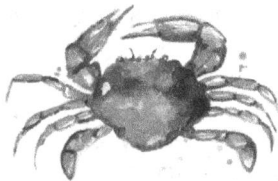

Pancreatic Cancer

What Is Pancreatic Cancer?

The pancreas makes enzymes to help digest food, and it is the source of insulin. It lies at the back of the abdomen, so when cancer develops, it does not usually become apparent until it has been growing for some time. There is no lump, and pain only occurs late after it has spread to the nerves and muscles near the back. It does not often block neighboring structures, such as the bile duct, and cause jaundice, until it is well-established.

As a result, by the time it is diagnosed, it is usually beyond cure. Although prevention is not always possible, there are a number of factors that we know predispose to its occurrence. By avoiding these, the possibility of getting this disease is reduced.

Who Gets Pancreatic Cancer?

Pancreatic cancer is the eighth most common cancer in the world, being more common in Western countries. The rate of occurrence in high-income countries is about three times that of low-income countries. In the US, it is the fourth most common cause of cancer death. While some cases occur as a result of inherited genes, many occur as a result of our lifestyle. In particular, people who smoke, those who are overweight, those who do not do much physical exercise, and those who drink a lot of alcohol are more likely to develop pancreatic cancer.

Preventing Pancreatic Cancer

Smoking

Cigarette smoking predisposes to pancreatic cancer and it has been estimated that one in four cases of pancreatic cancer occurs as a result of smoking. Smoking doubles a person's chances of getting the disease. When a smoker stops, over the next two years, the increased risk of getting pancreatic cancer is halved, and by fifteen years the risk is no different than nonsmokers.

Excess Body Fat

Being overweight or obese increases the risk of developing pancreatic cancer. Someone who is obese, as defined by a BMI over 30, has a 50 percent increased chance of developing pancreatic cancer. This applies to all methods of measuring excess body fat, be it by BMI, waist circumference, or waist-hip ratio. To put things in perspective, being obese increases the likelihood of developing pancreatic cancer from one in sixty-five (in a Western population) to about one in forty-five.

Physical Exercise

Even in people who are overweight, moderate physical activity on a regular basis can significantly reduce the pancreatic cancer risk. If you cannot lose weight, at least exercise regularly, as this will give some protection.

Alcohol

Drinking small amounts of alcohol probably does little harm to the pancreas, but once a level of three or more drinks of alcohol is reached, there is an increase in pancreatic cancer risk. Pancreatic cancer is also known to be associated with the condition of chronic pancreatitis, and the commonest cause of this is a heavy alcohol intake.

Diet

Whether diet plays a part in pancreatic cancer development is not certain. There is some evidence that a healthy diet, rich in fresh fruits, vegetables, whole grains, milk, and unsaturated oils, and low in saturated fats, alcohol, and added sugar, has a protective effect.

To Prevent Pancreatic Cancer

- Limit alcohol consumption.
- Be physically active.
- Don't smoke.
- Lose excess fat.
- Eat a healthy diet.

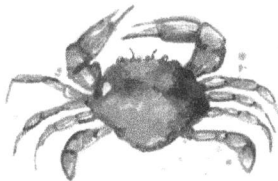

The Female Cancers

Breast Cancer
Ovarian Cancer
Uterine Cancer

Breast Cancer

What Is Breast Cancer?

The most common form of breast cancer is what we call epithelial cancer. The breast ducts and glands are lined by a layer of cells called epithelium, and this is where most breast cancers start. The normal growth of these cells is controlled by many factors but include the hormonal environment, so they grow or regress as the body needs them, such as during breastfeeding.

When they become cancerous, they grow in an uncontrolled manner so initially they form a lump, and later cells can break off and move through either the lymphatic system or the blood to spread to other parts of the body. There are a number of variants of the cancer, including ductal, lobular, tubular, or mucinous cancers, and these relate to how the cells appear in a microscope.

Getting breast cancer usually means surgery, radiation therapy, and often chemotherapy. It is one of the most curable cancers. With treatment, only about 10 percent of those who develop the disease are not still alive and well ten years after diagnosis. In recent decades, there has been improved awareness, early diagnosis, and better treatments of breast cancer, and these have all contributed to the improved survival.

Who Gets Breast Cancer?

Breast cancer is one of the commonest of cancers. In Western societies, as many as one in eight women will get it at some stage in their lives. In Asian countries, about one in sixteen women will be affected.

Because breast cells are under the control of the hormonal environment, it is not surprising that the occurrence of breast cancer is influenced by hormonal factors. It is more common in women who have an early menarche, a late menopause, have no or few babies or have their first child late in life, those who do not breastfeed, and in women who take hormones. Other factors, such as obesity, diet, and exercise, also play a part and even these might act by influencing hormone levels.

There are a number of inherited genetic mutations that increase breast cancer risk, such as BRCA1 and BRAC2. Women with these mutations have at least a one in two likelihood of getting breast cancer. Breast cancer is not restricted to women; men can also get it, but it is much less frequent and in men it is more likely to be associated with a genetic mutation such as BRCA1 or BRAC2.

Preventing Breast Cancer

Hormone Replacement Therapy (HRT).

At menopause, the ovaries cease to make estrogen and blood levels fall. This accounts for the flushes, sweats, sleep deprivation, and mood changes that can accompany menopause. It also results in increased bone loss and so predisposes to osteoporosis. Taking estrogens overcomes most of these problems. However, taking estrogens stimulates the uterus and predisposes it to cancer. This is prevented by adding a progestin. Consequently, unless a woman has had a hysterectomy, hormone replacement therapy is given as a combination of estrogen and progestin.

While HRT helps menopausal symptoms, it does have a downside. It can cause breast cancer. Once this became known in the 1990s, many women stopped taking HRT and a graph of breast cancer incidence over this time shows a corresponding drop in breast cancer occurrence.

The relationship between taking hormones and breast cancer is not simple, and some aspects are contradictory. Taking combined HRT, estrogen plus the progestin to protect the uterus, definitely increases breast cancer risk. However, those women who have had a hysterectomy and take estrogen-alone HRT do not have this increase in breast cancer. Note that the hormones given during in vitro fertilization (IVF) do not result in any increase in breast cancer.

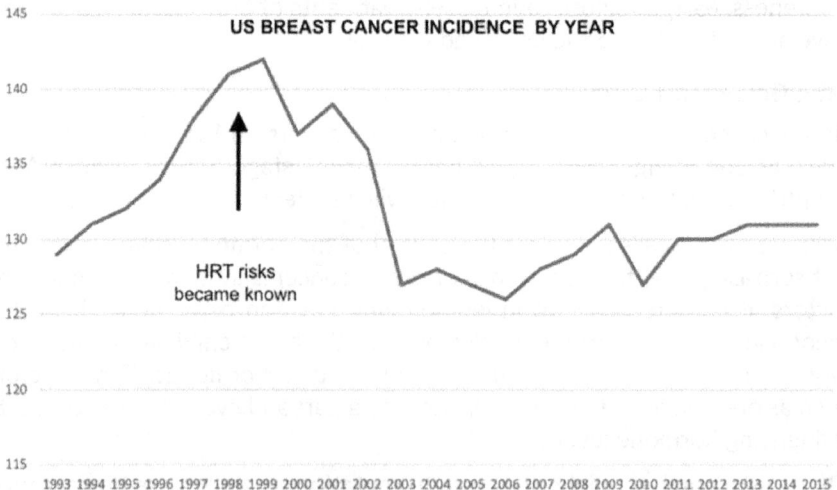

This graph shows the incidence of breast cancer in the US by year. There was a steady rise until 1998, probably due to increased detection from mammographic screening and increasing HRT use. About this time, the results of the Women's Health Initiative trial of HRT became available, which showed that HRT increased both breast cancer and heart disease. As a result, there was a 38 percent reduction in HRT use with twenty million fewer HRT prescriptions written. Breast cancer rates dropped dramatically and have plateaued since.

Oral and Intrauterine Hormonal Contraceptives

Oral contraceptives contain a progestin to suppress ovulation, and some also contain an estrogen. Intrauterine or implanted hormonal contraceptives also contain a progestin. In 1995, a study was commenced of the entire female population of Denmark who were ages fifteen to forty-nine at the time, totaling 1.8 million women. They were followed for the next eleven years and the contraceptive use of the 11,519 women who developed breast cancer during this time was compared to those who did not get breast cancer.

Current or recent users of hormonal contraception had an increased risk of breast cancer. For those who used it for a year or less, the risk was less than a 10 percent increase, but this increased steadily with increasing duration of use. For women who used hormonal contraception for ten or more years, there was a nearly 40 percent increase in risk.

However, for a young person using contraception, the risk is not as big as it sounds. For example, for a forty-year-old, someone who might have been on the OCP for many years, the chances of developing breast cancer in the next ten years is one in sixty-nine and a 40 percent increase in risk is still only a one in fifty possibility.

The risk persisted to some extent five years after stopping the hormonal contraception, although at a lower level. Risk was also increased in women who used progestin-only intrauterine contraceptive systems. The researchers estimated that for every 7,690 women using hormonal contraception for a year, there would be one extra breast cancer.

Excess Body Fat

Obese, postmenopausal women have a significantly higher risk of developing breast cancer, and once treated, they have an increased chance of recurrence of the cancer. This has been proven in more than 150 research studies. It is an estrogen effect.

Fat cells contain an enzyme called aromatase and this enzyme converts precursors in the blood to estrogen. The more body fat, the more estrogen. This is not a factor in obese, premenopausal women. For overweight, postmenopausal women (BMI 25–30), there is a 50 percent increased breast cancer risk, and if obese (BMI >30), the risk is doubled (100 percent increase).

This increased risk is particularly marked in those women who gained weight once they entered menopause. For overweight and obese women, this increase in risk is reversible. Studies have shown that by losing weight, breast cancer risk similarly diminishes. One study showed that when obese women underwent bariatric surgery, they halved their chances of getting breast cancer.

Physical Activity

Women who are physically inactive have an increased chance of developing breast cancer, with the converse being true: physically active women have a lower breast cancer risk. This has been examined in numerous studies involving tens of thousands of women. In general, when those women in the highest bracket of physical exercise are compared to those in the lowest, they have a 10 percent reduction in breast cancer risk. This is particularly so for postmenopausal women.

Some studies have tried to determine just how much exercise is needed. It would seem that breast cancer risk is reduced by 3 percent for every seven MET hours per week. These figures relate to all forms of physical activity, including occupational and recreational.

Vigorous physical activity has been looked at as a separate factor and the results again show benefit in exercise. Here the benefit was greatest for premenopausal women. It was estimated that for every thirty minutes of vigorous physical exercise per day, the breast cancer risk diminished by 10 percent.

There are several mechanisms by which physical activity could reduce breast cancer risk. Physical activity improves insulin sensitivity, it reduces estrogen levels in postmenopausal women, and improves immunity.

Diet

A healthy diet, be it vegetarian, Mediterranean, or any diet with a largely vegetable base, is associated with a lower chance of getting many cancers, breast cancer included.

Two pooled analyses of smaller studies that involved tens of thousands of women have shown that vegetable consumption, and in particular non-starchy vegetables, reduced breast cancer by up to 20 percent. It is necessary to eat 200–300 gm (two to three servings) per day to achieve this. The benefit from vegetable consumption was for the more aggressive estrogen-receptor negative type of breast cancer.

Similar studies looked at beta-carotene consumption and beta-carotene levels in the blood. A high beta-carotene consumption or blood level was associated with a 10–20 percent reduction in breast cancer risk, and again this was predominantly for estrogen-receptor negative cancers.

Blood levels seemed to be more important than dietary consumption. The amount measured in the blood did not correlate well with the amount eaten, suggesting that absorption and metabolism, also food processing and cooking methods, were just as important as the amount eaten. Beta-carotene is found in a wide variety of fruits and vegetables, and there are numerous mechanisms by which they might protect against cancer.

Most studies have shown that calcium consumption is protective for breast cancer, with one pooled analysis showing a more than 10 percent reduction in breast cancer risk per 300 mg of calcium consumed. Calcium plays an important role in regulating cell function and growth, and potentially is important in controlling cell proliferation.

There is some evidence that phytoestrogens, derived from either soy or the outer coating of cereals, can help protect against breast cancer.

Alcohol

There have been at least sixteen large, well-conducted studies of alcohol consumption and premenopausal breast cancer, and at least thirty-four studies on postmenopausal breast cancer. Virtually every one of them has shown that alcohol consumption increases a woman's risk of getting breast cancer.

For premenopausal women, every 10 gm of alcohol consumed on average per day results in a 5 percent increase in breast cancer risk. For postmenopausal women, this is closer to 10 percent per 10 gm consumed.

Thus, up to one alcoholic drink per day has only a small increase in breast cancer risk. Once this becomes two or more on average each day, the risk significantly increases. There are multiple mechanisms by which alcohol could influence the development of breast cancer, one being that alcohol is metabolized in the breast to acetaldehyde, which is a carcinogen.

Radiation

If a young breast is exposed to radiation, it is more likely to develop breast cancer. The breast is most sensitive to radiation between the ages of ten and fourteen, but it remains still susceptible until about age forty-five. We know this from the survivors of the atomic bomb blasts. In addition, we know that young women might have an increased risk of developing breast cancer after receiving radiation therapy as a child for Hodgkin's lymphoma.

Some are given what is called mantle radiation therapy, where X-rays are beamed into the chest to treat the cancerous lymph nodes. Some of the inner breast can be irradiated during this treatment. Although the treatment can cure the Hodgkin's disease, the breast needs to be carefully monitored on account of the small but definite increased breast cancer risk in this area.

Mammograms use radiation to produce an image of the breast and so detect breast cancer. They are commonly used both as a screening tool in healthy women who do not have any breast symptoms, and in women with a breast lump or other symptom to try to determine their nature. While there is considerable benefit in having mammograms, they are not completely harmless.

Radiation can increase the risk of cancer developing. In particular, radiation is more damaging to young tissues, so the younger the exposure to radiation, the higher the risk. For example, if women were to have an annual mammogram from age twenty onward, it would probably result in more lives lost due to breast cancer than lives saved. This is an extreme example, but if you are young and your doctor recommends such a thing, decline.

By age forty-five, the breast tissues are much less susceptible to radiation damage and the risk of a mammogram causing cancer is small. There is no doubt that mammograms, when used appropriately, are valuable in the diagnosis of breast cancer. Screening programs vary from country to country, but a common approach is to start screening at forty-five to fifty, with films every two years. This will result in a reduction in deaths from breast cancer of about 20 percent.

Breastfeeding

Women who breastfeed have a lower risk of developing breast cancer, although this is a relatively minor factor. It has been estimated that for every six months of breastfeeding, breast cancer risk diminishes by 2 percent. This mainly relates to estrogen-receptor negative breast cancers.

Aspirin

The California Teachers Study followed 57,164 women, of whom 1,457 developed invasive breast cancer. This study showed that low-dose aspirin use was associated with a 16 percent reduction in breast cancer.

Disturbed Sleep Rhythm

Airline cabin attendants and night-time shift workers have at least a 50 percent increased risk of getting breast cancer, and nurses who regularly rotate from day to night shifts have a doubling of their risk. Research has shown that nocturnal light exposure suppresses melatonin, and low levels of this are associated with breast cancer risk.

Fertility

Women who do not have children have a significantly higher risk of developing breast cancer, and the more children, the lower the risk. Probably more important is the age at first pregnancy, with the younger a woman is when she has her first child, the lower the risk. This is something that might be beyond a woman's control. Infertility is a common problem, and social convention plays a big part in determining at what age a woman first gets pregnant.

Treat Precancerous Lesions

Sometimes a mammogram finds a precancerous lesion. The term "lesion" is commonly used in medicine and all it means is that there is something present that is not normal. In the breast, there are a number of lesions that, while harmless, if not treated might become a cancer. Examples are low-risk lesions, such as atypical ductal hyperplasia or a radial scar, or something at higher risk of turning into an invasive cancer such as ductal carcinoma in situ.

These lesions are called precancerous lesions, and while some will become a cancer, in a lot of cases, they will not. In time, about half of all cases of high-grade duct carcinoma in situ will become an invasive cancer. There is no way of knowing which will, or will not, end up as an invasive cancer, and so in most cases they are removed, and this is normally just a small procedure.

To Prevent Breast Cancer

- Limit alcohol consumption.
- Aim for at least thirty minutes of physical exercise each day.
- Lose excess fat.
- Eat a diet rich in fruits and vegetables, calcium, and phytoestrogens.
- Keep HRT use to the minimum duration you can manage.
- Remove precancerous lesions found on screening.
- Breastfeed, if possible.

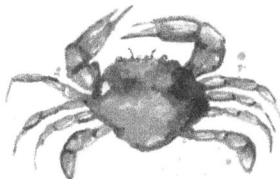

Ovarian Cancer

What Is Ovarian Cancer?

The ovaries are situated in the female pelvis, adjacent to the fallopian tubes. They produce eggs and are the source of hormone production in women before menopause. Cancer occurs mainly in the outer lining and is called epithelial ovarian cancer. It can also start in the fallopian tubes, or even the lining of the abdomen, the peritoneum.

As the ovaries are hidden deep in the pelvis, there is plenty of room for them to grow—think about the space a baby needs to develop when in the uterus—so a cancer can become large and spread before anyone is aware of its presence.

Who Gets Ovarian Cancer?

Worldwide, there are about a quarter of a million cases of ovarian cancer each year. It is the seventh most common cancer in women, being more common in women in Western countries. The overall rate for women in the UK and Europe is about 11–12/100,000 women per year. In the US, it is 8/100,000, while in South America, Africa, and China, the rate is only 4–5/100,000.

Ovarian cancer mostly occurs in older women, after menopause. Some occur as a result of an inherited genetic mutation, BRCA1 or BRAC2. These genetic mutations can also cause breast cancer. As with breast cancer, women who get ovarian cancer as a result of this genetic mutation tend to get their cancer at an earlier age.

There are many similarities with breast cancer. Ovarian cancer is more common in women who start their periods early, have a late menopause, do not have children or have them late in life, and who do not breastfeed. These features all suggest a hormonal relationship.

Preventing Ovarian Cancer

Oral Contraceptive Pill (OCP)

For every five years of OCP use, the risk of developing ovarian cancer reduces by 20 percent, so women who have taken the OCP for fifteen years have at least halved their chances of getting the disease. This protective effect lasts for decades after stopping the OCP, with some benefit twenty years later.

Preventive Surgery

Women who have inherited a BRCA1 genetic mutation have a one in two chance of developing ovarian cancer, and a one in four chance if they have the BRCA2 mutation. With such a high risk, consideration should be given to the risk reduction surgery of removing the ovaries and tubes once childbearing is complete. This is normally a keyhole surgery. Taking an oral estrogen can replace the loss of hormone production.

Breastfeeding

Women who have breastfed their children have a lower risk of getting ovarian cancer, and those who fed for a total of twelve months or more have a 30 percent lower risk. Even breastfeeding for six months provides some degree of protection.

Excess Body Fat

Like many other cancers, having too much fat increases the risk of getting ovarian cancer. This increase in risk is small and seems to only be an effect at the higher levels of obesity.

Soy Consumption

Soy is rich in phytoestrogens, or plant-based estrogens. These natural estrogens are thought to compete with the body's own estrogen for hormone receptors in various organs. Because they are weaker, they could act as a natural antiestrogen, by blocking the body's own estrogen from the receptors. A number of studies have suggested that women with a high consumption of soy have a reduced incidence of ovarian cancer.

To Prevent Ovarian Cancer

If You Have a BRCA Gene Mutation
- Consider preventive tube and ovary removal, once childbearing is finished

If You Are Taking an OCP
- Taking the OCP, or having taken it in the past, reduces ovarian cancer risk.

For All Women
- Breastfeed, if there is the opportunity.
- Lose excess fat.
- Have soy in your diet.

Uterine Cancer

What Is Uterine Cancer?

There are two distinct types of cancer of the uterus. Cancer of the endometrium (body of the uterus) and cancer of the cervix of the uterus. These have different causes, so the changes we can do to prevent them are different.

Cancer of the Endometrium

The endometrium is the lining of the main body of the uterus. It is here that a fertilized egg implants. If this doesn't happen, it is shed each month, resulting in bleeding. After menopause, it is still present, but in an atrophied state. The uterus is under the control of the body's hormones, estrogen and progesterone. In a premenopausal woman, each month these hormones prepare the endometrial lining for the possibility of receiving an egg.

Cancer can develop in the cells of this layer, and this is more likely to occur if there is a high level of hormones in the blood. This is predominantly a problem in a postmenopausal woman because the body can no longer make progesterone to balance any estrogen. Excess estrogen might occur from taking HRT or being produced by fat cells. Such a situation makes the uterine endometrium prone to cancer.

Cancer of the Cervix of the Uterus

The cervix is the lower end of the uterus that protrudes into the vagina. It has a small opening to allow the entry of sperm and to prevent the premature release of a fetus. During childbirth, it stretches enormously to let the baby out. Being more external than the body of the uterus, it is more exposed to factors that can cause cancer. In the case of the cervix of the uterus, it is infection with the HPV virus that is most likely to turn the cells cancerous.

Who Gets Uterine Cancer?

Cancer of the Endometrium

Endometrial cancer is the sixth most common cancer in women, with more than half a million cases each year. It is most common in high-income countries, being about three times more common in North America and Europe than in Africa. As with cancer of the breast or ovary, it is more common in women who have not had children and in those who have a natural late menopause.

The majority of these cancers occur after menopause, and because the main symptom of postmenopausal bleeding occurs at an early stage and is obvious, they tend to be diagnosed and treated early. As a result, most women who develop endometrial cancer are cured by treatment.

A common factor in women who develop uterine endometrial cancer is an excess of estrogen stimulation. There are a number of sources of estrogen stimulation, apart from the obvious one of taking estrogen hormone replacement therapy (HRT) to alleviate menopausal symptoms.

In particular, after menopause a source of estrogen is the fat cells. These contain an enzyme called aromatase that makes estrogen. Women who have excess body fat have more estrogen.

Another source of estrogen stimulation of the endometrium is tamoxifen, a drug commonly taken by women who have had breast cancer to help prevent recurrence. While tamoxifen acts as an antiestrogen on breast cells and breast cancer cells, on the uterus it paradoxically acts like an estrogen. In time this estrogenic stimulation of the endometrium can lead to endometrial cancer. This is a rare occurrence and the number of lives saved from breast cancer by tamoxifen far outweighs any lost to endometrial cancer.

Cancer of the Cervix of the Uterus

Cancer of the cervix of the uterus is a common and sometimes lethal disease, the fourth most common cancer of women. Its occurrence is almost entirely due to human papillomavirus (HPV) infection. The HPV virus can be detected in almost 100 percent of cases.

Most developed countries have screening programs in place for early detection of cervical cancer, or even the preliminary changes that can be seen in the cells before a cancer has fully developed. The prevention, screening, and treatment of cervical cancer is rapidly changing because vaccines, to effectively prevent HPV infection, are now available. There is the possibility of virtually eliminating cervical cancer by HPV immunization.

Preventing Cancer of the Endometrium

Avoid Estrogen-Only HRT

Women who have not had a hysterectomy and who use estrogen-only HRT, that is, not combined with a progestin, have a marked increased risk of getting endometrial cancer. The longer the use, the higher the risk. Even after one year, the preliminary changes of endometrial hyperplasia are present in many women.

By balancing the estrogen with a progestin in the HRT, this effect on the uterus is negated. The use of estrogen-only HRT is only safe in women who have had their uterus removed.

Low-dose vaginal estrogen used topically appears to be safe but should still be used with caution.

Use of Hormonal Contraceptives

Hormonal contraceptives contain a progestin. In the oral contraceptive pill (OCP) this is either in combination with an estrogen or is a progestin alone. There are also progestin containing implants under the skin for contraception, or in an intrauterine device (IUD) contraceptive. All of these protect against uterine cancer.

After five years of OCP use, the risk is diminished by about 25 percent and the benefit increases with increasing duration of use. Furthermore, once the progestin-containing contraception is stopped, the protection persists for decades.

A study from Finland found that women who had a progestin containing IUD halved their risk of getting endometrial cancer. While you would not normally take the OCP or use a progestin-IUD just to prevent uterine cancer, it does provide some reassurance for those who are using them, also for those who have used them in the past.

Excess Body Fat

Fat cells are a source of estrogen. Once menopause has been reached, this estrogen is no longer balanced by progestin. This allows it to stimulate the endometrium. As a result, having excess body fat is one of the most important risk factors for developing endometrial cancer. Compared to a woman with a BMI in the normal range of less than 25, someone with a BMI of more than 35 is almost five times more likely to develop endometrial cancer.

Physical Activity

Physically active women are less likely to develop endometrial cancer than inactive women. This applies to the physical activity gained during an active type of occupation and to women who intentionally exercise regularly.

Phytoestrogens

There is some suggestion from dietary studies that a diet rich in plant-derived estrogens, such as a soy-rich diet, might help protect against endometrial cancer, as soy is thought to be a natural antiestrogen.

Preventing Cervical Cancer of the Uterus

HPV Infection

Virtually all cancers of the cervix are associated with HPV infection, but not all HPV infections result in cervical cancer. It is believed that about 75–80 percent of sexually active adults will acquire HPV at some stage, but in most people the infection is transient. In some, however, the virus persists and damages the cells lining the cervix, so causing cancer.

This process takes a long time, perhaps as long as fifteen years. The process can be detected at an early stage, years before a cancer has developed. The cells can show signs of cervical intraepithelial neoplasia (CIN), something seen on microscopic examination of a smear of cervical cells, known as a Papanicolaou smear. If treated at this stage, the cancer might be prevented. Why the virus persists in some people is not known but this situation is more common with a deficient immune system, such as in someone with HIV.

There are about forty different strains of HPV, but only some of them cause cervical cancer. Vaccines have been developed against most of these cancer-causing strains and result in effective immunity. If given before a person becomes sexually active, that person will not get an HPV infection and so will not go on and develop cervical cancer.

Many countries have organized vaccination programs for HPV prevention. A review of data from Scotland showed that girls immunized with a bivalent vaccine, an early form of vaccination for HPV, had an 89 percent reduction in high-grade CIN, the precursor of cervical cancer, or cervical cancer itself, by age twenty. Vaccination at twelve to thirteen years was much more effective than vaccination at seventeen. In theory, cervical cancer can be largely eliminated by vaccination, although this depends on the rate of immunization take-up.

A male can become infected from intercourse with an infected woman and while he obviously does not get cervical cancer, if he has intercourse with other women, he can infect them and so the disease is spread. This has resulted in arguments about who should be immunized, should it just be girls, or should boys also be immunized? Just vaccinating girls will prevent cervical cancer, but if boys are vaccinated too, the spread of the virus can be eliminated. Furthermore, males also get diseases from HPV, so these could also be prevented if males are vaccinated. These include cancer of the anus, penis, and oropharynx, in addition to genital warts.

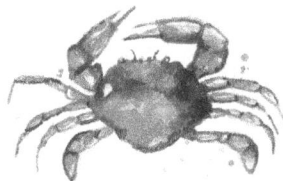

To Prevent Cancer of the Endometrium

- Lose excess fat.
- If HRT is to be used, estrogen should be combined with a progestin.
- Hormonal contraceptives are beneficial.
- Aim for at least thirty minutes of physical exercise each day.
- Eat a diet rich in phytoestrogens.

To Prevent Cancer of the Cervix of the Uterus

- Encourage HPV vaccination of all children.
- Treat CIN lesions found on screening.

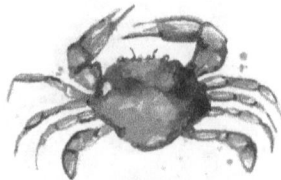

The Male Cancers

Prostate Cancer

Testicular Cancer

Prostate Cancer

What Is Prostate Cancer?

The prostate gland is a walnut-sized organ situated at the outlet of the bladder in males. Its function is to produce and eject fluid at the time of ejaculation. This fluid surrounds and protects the sperm. When a cancer develops in the lining of the gland, the gland enlarges. The first thing that happens is the flow of urine becomes weaker. The prostate surrounds the urethra, the tube by which urine passes out of the bladder, obstructing flow.

Unfortunately, prostate cancer can spread, usually to the bones, before it starts blocking off the flow of urine, so it might not be diagnosed until it is too late for a cure. This has led to the widespread use of the prostate-specific antigen (PSA) test, a blood test to detect the cancer before it has spread to the bones or other parts of the body.

Who Gets Prostate Cancer?

The prostate is a common site for cancer to develop. In many countries, it is the commonest form of cancer in men. It is expected that before long, prostate cancer will be the commonest cancer in men worldwide, overtaking lung cancer. There are nearly two million cases diagnosed worldwide each year. It is more common in Western populations and men in Australia, Europe, and North America are twenty-five times more likely to get prostate cancer than men in less well-developed nations. In the US, about one in six men will be diagnosed with prostate cancer at some stage in their lives.

The number of people known to have prostate cancer has increased in recent years for several reasons. First, it becomes more common as we age, and the world's population is living longer. Second, less well-developed countries are improving their standard of living. As this happens, the rate of prostate cancer increases. Third, it is being detected more commonly due to PSA screening becoming more widely used. This does not mean there are more cases, it just means we know about what might have been previously undetected cancers.

If present in a man, the BRCA2 gene mutation makes him more likely to develop prostate cancer. This is the same mutation that predisposes women to breast and ovarian cancer. There are a number of other inherited genetic defects that have been identified that can also lead to prostate cancer. As many as 10 percent of all prostate cancers run in families, and many of these are due to an abnormal gene being passed on, from the mother or the father.

Preventing Prostate Cancer

Excess Body Fat

Having excess body fat increases the chances of not only getting prostate cancer, but it also increases the chances of dying from prostate cancer. For every five points of BMI above normal, there is a 5 percent increase in the risk of getting prostate cancer and an 11 percent increase in the chances of dying from prostate cancer.

The mode of action of excess body fat is most likely though insulin and IGF-1. Both of these have been shown to be associated with increased prostate cancer risk and are known to promote the growth of cancer cells. Getting rid of excess body fat is important in reducing prostate cancer risk.

Smoking

While it is not clear if smoking increases the chances of getting prostate cancer, there is no doubt that it increases the chances of recurrence after treatment of prostate cancer, and death from the cancer. The more cigarettes smoked, the greater the risk. If you have had prostate cancer and smoke, then stopping will improve your chances of surviving the cancer.

Diet

Dairy Products. There is evidence that men who have a lot of dairy products in their diet have a higher risk of getting prostate cancer. For every 400 gm eaten daily, the risk increases by 6 percent. It is thought that this might be related to the calcium in dairy as calcium can affect prostate cell growth. Dairy consumption is also associated with higher IGF-1 levels.

Phytoestrogens. Phytoestrogens are plant-derived estrogens, mainly from soy, and it is thought they might reduce prostate cancer risk. There have not been a lot of studies in humans but what there are, suggest some protection from prostate cancer.

Lycopene. One prospective cohort study of over 50,000 men showed that dietary lycopene, an antioxidant found in tomatoes, might reduce prostate cancer occurrence and deaths

Coffee. Coffee has been shown to be protective for a number of cancers. With prostate cancer, the more coffee drunk each day, the lower the risk of dying from the disease.

To Prevent Prostate Cancer

- Lose excess fat.
- Do not smoke.
- Drink coffee.

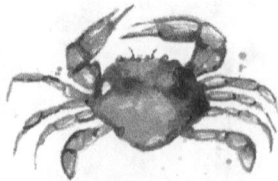

Testicular Cancer

What Is Testicular Cancer?

The usual form of testicular cancer is what we call a germ cell tumor, where the reproductive cells in the testis, those that form sperm, undergo malignant change. Variants of germ cell tumors include seminoma or teratoma of the testis. They become apparent when a painless lump appears in the testis.

Who Gets Testicular Cancer?

Testicular cancer is not common, with only about 75,000 case worldwide each year. It is a cancer that can be effectively treated, even when it has spread to other parts of the body, so most people who develop testicular cancer survive.

There is one particular group of men who are at higher risk of developing testicular cancer and that is those with what we call an undescended testis. The testes develop inside the abdomen. Normally, just before birth, the testes descend and pass through the abdominal wall into the scrotum.

In some men, this does not happen and one or both of the testes gets arrested in its descent and never reaches the scrotum. The risk of developing testicular cancer is five to ten times higher than men who have normally positioned testes. If the testes cannot be made to move into the scrotum by surgery, then it should be removed, rather than leave it inside the abdomen where it is at risk of becoming malignant.

Preventing Testicular Cancer

There is no evidence that having a vasectomy increases the risk of testicular cancer, although there is some evidence that heavy users of marijuana do have an increase in risk.

To Prevent Testicular Cancer

- Avoid heavy use of marijuana.
- Remove testes that have not descended.

Cancers of the Respiratory Tract

Nasopharyngeal Cancer

Cancers of the Larynx, Bronchi, and Lung

Mesothelioma

The respiratory tract enables us to get air into our lungs and breathe. It consists of a number of structures and any of these can development malignant change. The inhaled air first passes through the nose and nasopharynx, past the mouth (through which you can also take in air) into the larynx, where our voice box is situated. From there down the trachea to the bronchi, which are smaller breathing tubes. These lead into the lungs where inhaled oxygen is exchanged with carbon dioxide, which is then exhaled.

Nasopharyngeal Cancer

What Is Nasopharyngeal Cancer?

The nasopharynx is a narrow passage connected to, and immediately behind, the nose. Cancer that originates from the lining of this nasal passage is a squamous cell cancer. The majority are caused by viral infections. More than 90 percent of nasopharyngeal tumors from patients in China have Epstein-Barr virus (EBV) particles in them. Some, but less than 10 percent, have HPV particles, suggesting this virus is an alternative cause. In Western countries, EBV infection is also common but it rarely results in nasopharyngeal cancer. It is thought that the EBV is activated in Asia by a combination of factors, such as eating preserved foods, smoking, and perhaps a genetic predisposition, resulting in DNA damage.

Who Gets Nasopharyngeal Cancer?

Nasopharyngeal cancer is common in southern China and Hong Kong, where the incidence is about twenty times that of Europe and the US. It is more common in males and tends to occur in midlife. Worldwide, nearly 100,000 cases occur annually with a high mortality.

Preventing Nasopharyngeal Cancer

Vaccination

While there is no vaccine or treatment for EBV infection at present, there are active attempts to develop a vaccine. There is a vaccine to prevent HPV. Many countries have HPV immunization programs designed to eradicate cervical cancer, which might help with HPV particles found in nasopharyngeal cancer.

Diet

Salt-preserved and pickled foods contain high levels of nitrosamines and these can be carcinogenic. These foods are commonly eaten in the high-risk areas of southern China. It is thought that they activate the EBV virus to cause nasopharyngeal cancer, so should be avoided.

Smoking and Alcohol

Use of alcohol and tobacco are more common in people with nasopharyngeal cancer. They are thought to activate the EBV.

To Prevent Nasopharyngeal Cancer

- Avoid salt-preserved and pickled foods.
- Do not smoke.
- Limit alcohol.
- Encourage HPV vaccination

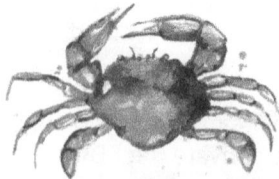

Cancers of the Larynx, Bronchi, and Lung

What Is Lung Cancer?

Although the larynx, bronchi, and lungs are anatomically different, they are all part of the respiratory tract. When they develop cancer, there is a common cause—smoking. Inhaled smoke travels down these airways and can damage the lining layer of cells. This includes secondhand smoke exhaled by someone else in the room. In some people, these cellular changes go on to become cancer. The cause and preventive measures are the same as for lung cancer.

Who Gets Lung Cancer?

Worldwide, there are about two million cases of lung cancer each year. For men, it is the commonest cancer, and for women, the third most common cancer. It is becoming less common in some countries, because fewer people are smoking. For example, in Australia, the percentage of male smokers has reduced from 43 percent in 1976 to 16 percent in 2016. As a result, annual lung cancer rates have fallen from about 85 to 55 cases per 100,000 population over this time and are still falling.

In the US, deaths from lung cancer in men have fallen by 45 percent between 1990 and 2015, again associated with a reduction in smoking. In many countries, the number of smokers remains high, such as in China and Russia, where about 45–50 percent of men smoke. In all countries, women smoke less, but the rate of women smoking is increasing, and, as a result, their lung cancer incidence is rising.

Not everyone who gets lung cancer is a smoker. For men, about 15 percent have never smoked, while for women, 50 percent of lung cancer cases are nonsmokers. This does vary from region to region with 20 percent of US women with lung cancer never having smoked to 60–80 percent in Asia.

The reasons nonsmokers get lung cancer is not altogether clear, but it is likely that passive smoking, inhaling smoke exhaled by someone else, is important. Inhaling atmospheric pollution and inhaling naturally occurring radon gas are also causative factors.

Preventing Lung Cancer

Smoking

If you have never smoked, do not start, as smoking is the main cause of lung cancer. If you are a smoker, then stop. The risk depends on how heavily and for how long someone has smoked cigarettes, but a long-term smoker has a thirty times increased chance of getting lung cancer. A lifetime heavy smoker has almost a one in three probability of developing the disease.

When a smoker quits, a reduction in lung cancer risk starts to be seen after five years. If the smoker has managed not to smoke for fifteen years, the risk has reduced by 80–90 percent. Even people who quit after being treated for lung cancer have a better chance of surviving. Cigar and pipe smoking are also associated with an increased lung cancer risk, although this is less than with cigarette smoking. It is too early to know if smoking electronic cigarettes is associated with lung cancer.

Passive smoking, breathing in smoke exhaled by a smoker, is also associated with lung cancer. While the intensity of smoke is less, and it is a less common cause of lung cancer, for nonsmokers, it does pose a significant risk. It has been estimated that up to 25 percent of all lung cancers that occur in nonsmokers are a result of passive smoking.

A Japanese study estimated that a nonsmoker who lives with someone who smokes doubles their risk of getting lung cancer. Children exposed to passive smoking are at greater risk than being exposed to passive smoking later in life.

Avoid Air Pollution

People who live in areas of high atmospheric pollution are at increased risk of getting lung cancer. This is particularly so in regard to diesel fumes where nonsmokers are 30 percent more likely to get the disease than someone who is not exposed to this air pollution. Long-term exposure to even low levels of air pollution also increases lung cancer risk. If you have a choice, live away from busy roads and high-pollution cities.

Avoid Radon in Buildings

Radon is a naturally occurring radioactive gas, and people who inhale high levels are at increased risk of developing lung cancer. Radon can accumulate in buildings that are not well-ventilated and that are built in areas where the soil is rich in uranium, thorium, and radium. In the US, it is the second most common cause of lung cancer.

Diet

There is good evidence that a diet rich in vegetables and fruits, and low in red meat, lowers the risk of developing lung cancer. In quantitative terms, for every 100 gm of fruits and vegetables eaten, the risk of getting lung cancer diminishes by 6–8 percent, so a large fruit-and-vegetable eater might expect a 10–15 percent lower chance of getting lung cancer, especially in a smoker. For every 100 gm of red meat eaten per day, the risk of getting lung cancer increases by 20 percent.

Beta-Carotene

Randomized controlled trials (RCTs) are important in proving if some preventative measures work. Postulated biological mechanisms and some non-RCT research had suggested that beta-carotene might prevent lung cancer. Trials were set up in the expectation that giving beta-carotene supplements to smokers would reduce their risk of getting lung cancer. The converse was true.

Those who took high-dose beta-carotene supplements had a 20 percent higher rate of getting lung cancer. While dietary sourced beta-carotene might be protective, supplementary beta-carotene in high doses can promote the development of lung cancer and should be avoided in current and past smokers.

To Prevent Lung Cancer

- Do not smoke.
- Do not breathe secondhand smoke.
- Avoid air pollution.
- Avoid breathing radon gas with good home ventilation.
- Eat fruits and vegetables but reduce red meat.
- Do not take high-dose beta-carotene supplements.

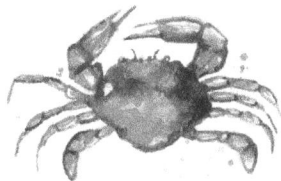

Mesothelioma

What Is Mesothelioma?

Mesothelioma is a form of cancer that develops in the lining of the lung, known as the pleura. Occasionally, it can develop elsewhere in the body, such as in the lining of the abdomen, known as the peritoneum. It is rare to survive mesothelioma.

Who Gets Mesothelioma?

Nearly every case of mesothelioma occurs as a result of asbestos exposure. In most cases, there has been a known episode, or multiple episodes, of exposure to asbestos. It is likely that in other cases, there has been some inadvertent exposure.

Not everyone exposed to asbestos will get mesothelioma; workers in the asbestos industry having a one in ten chance of getting the disease. Often it is not until thirty or more years after the asbestos exposure that the mesothelioma appears. The greater the exposure, the higher the chance of getting mesothelioma, although for some people even a brief exposure can trigger the disease.

Preventing Mesothelioma

Asbestos exposure is to be avoided at all costs. This can be difficult, as asbestos was used widely in the building industry where it was valuable for its insulating qualities. Many older buildings have asbestos in them. Some soils are high in asbestos and in other situations, old building materials with asbestos in them might have been dumped near habitation.

Because of our awareness of the dangers of asbestos, public health measures have reduced asbestos exposure, so in some countries the incidence of mesothelioma is falling. Worryingly, some developed countries still allow the use of asbestos in certain industries.

To Prevent Mesothelioma

- Avoid all contact with asbestos

Cancers of the Urinary Tract

Renal Cancer

Bladder Cancer

The body filters blood through the kidney, and excess fluid and unwanted substances become urine. The urine passes into what is called the renal pelvis, adjacent to the kidney, then down a long tube called the ureter to the bladder, where it is stored. When the bladder is full, we get the urge to empty the urine and it comes out through a short tube called the urethra.

Renal Cancer

What Is Renal Cancer?

The body uses the urinary system to get rid of unwanted substances. Some people think of these as "toxins," although most of what is excreted is just excess of body needs. For example, if we eat too much salt, the body excretes the excess in the urine, or if we eat a lot of oranges, the vitamin C in excess of what the body needs is excreted in the urine.

In someone with poor kidney function, substances can build up and become toxic. The body also gets rid of some drugs in the urine. An example of this was during World War II when penicillin was in short supply. The urine of soldiers being treated with penicillin was collected and the excreted penicillin was extracted and reused!

Cancer of the kidney is called renal cancer, or renal cell cancer. Renal cancer is uncommon, probably because the urine passes through quickly and so there is little time for contact. The lining of the bladder is more prone to cancer as urine, containing potentially toxic substances, stays there until the bladder is emptied.

Who Gets Renal Cancer?

Renal cancer is the twelfth most common cancer worldwide, with a few hundred thousand cases reported each year. It is more common in men and, like most cancers, becomes more common as we get older. It is more common in well-developed countries, such as the US and European nations, and it is expected to become more common worldwide as poorer countries develop.

Preventing Renal Cancer

Smoking

People who smoke are 50 percent more likely to get renal cancer than nonsmokers. This risk drops considerably after stopping smoking.

Excess Body Fat

Every study of excess body fat and renal cancer, and there have been more than twenty, has shown that having excess fat increases the risk of getting renal cancer. This is regardless of how body fat is measured, be it by BMI, girth measurements, or waist-hip ratio. The risk increases progressively with increase in excess fat, and for every five points of BMI above normal, the risk increases by 30 percent. For someone who is obese, this equates to an increase in lifetime risk of developing renal cancer from about one in eighty to one in sixty-two.

Alcohol

Drinking alcohol has been shown in many studies to reduce the risk of getting renal cancer, both in light and in moderate drinkers. It has been estimated that for every 10 gm of alcohol consumed each day, the risk reduces by 8 percent. It does not matter what type of alcohol, beer, wine, or spirits, the benefit is there.

Why alcohol helps protect against renal cancer when it tends to be a cause of many other cancers is not fully understood, but it might relate to its diuretic effect, as the urine passes more quickly through the renal tract. Alcoholic drinks also contain some antioxidants that could have a protective effect.

To Prevent Renal Cancer

- Do not smoke.
- Lose excess body fat.
- Light and moderate drinking of alcohol is beneficial.

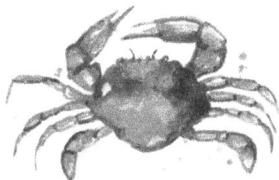

Bladder Cancer

What Is Bladder Cancer?

Bladder cancer occurs when the cells that line the bladder, known as the urothelium, undergo malignant change and so grow in an uncontrolled manner. It is sometimes called urothelial cancer and it can also occur in other parts of the urine excretion system, such as the renal pelvis, ureter, and urethra, but it is most common in the bladder. It is usually detected early, as these cancers bleed and blood is noticed in the urine.

Who Gets Bladder Cancer?

In men, bladder cancer is the ninth most common cancer worldwide. Most cases occur because potentially carcinogenic substances excreted in the urine spend time in the bladder in contact with the urothelium. This was first recognized as a problem in the 1950s, when aniline dyes, used in the textile industry, were found to be associated with a higher risk of bladder cancer among workers in that industry. These days, excreted metabolites from smoking are by far the most common cause of bladder cancer, although exposure to industrial chemicals is still a problem.

Preventing Bladder Cancer

Smoking

Smokers are about four times more likely to get bladder cancer than nonsmokers, and smoking accounts for 50 percent of all bladder cancers. The risk does diminish with time after stopping smoking, but former smokers are still at higher risk of getting bladder cancer. Being exposed to passive smoking is also associated with an increased chance of getting bladder cancer. Cigarette smoking is worse than cigar or pipe smoking.

Water

It is not surprising that people who drink a lot of water have a lower risk of getting bladder cancer, because the extra fluid dilutes any carcinogens in the urine and the bladder is emptied more frequently. One large cohort study showed that those who drank more than 2.5 liters (two-thirds of a gallon) of water each day had half the risk of getting bladder cancer compared to someone who drank less than 1.3 liters (one-third of a gallon) each day.

Avoid Toxins

Arsenic is known to occur in some drinking-water sources, particularly when ground water is drunk in areas where the soil is naturally high in arsenic compounds. This is mainly in Taiwan, where people who drank water from arsenic-contaminated wells had a tenfold to twentyfold increase in their risk of getting bladder cancer. Arsenic is known to be a carcinogen and when contaminated water is drunk, the arsenic is absorbed from the gut, then excreted by the kidneys and damages the bladder. This is now less common due to changes in drinking-water sources.

Workers in some industries are known to have a higher risk of bladder cancer. This is most likely due to toxins absorbed from the work environment. These industries include metal, leather, paint, rubber, and textile industries.

Diet

People who eat a lot of fresh fruits and vegetables have a lower risk of bladder cancer, but the benefit is small.

To Prevent Bladder Cancer

- Do not smoke.
- Do not breathe secondhand smoke.
- Drink plenty of water.
- Avoid environmental toxins, such as arsenic.
- Eat fruits and vegetables.

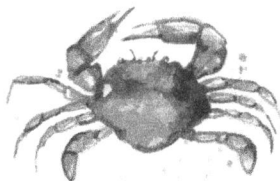

Skin Cancer

If older than fifty, with a skin color that is not naturally dark, and you spent your childhood in a sun-drenched country, such as Australia or the southern US states, the chances are you have sun-damaged skin and are at risk of developing skin cancer. You might have already had that experience.

The damage that sun exposure does to the skin of children was not recognized until the 1960s, and sunscreen use did not become widespread until the 1970s. All it takes is a few episodes of sunburn or seeking a tan by sunbaking or using a solarium, to damage the skin.

What Is Skin Cancer?

The outer layer of our skin is constantly regenerating from what is called the basal layer of cells. The old cells gradually work their way to the surface and are shed as dead cells. This layer of cells can be eighty cells thick, and these, together with a protein called keratin that is made by these cells, makes us waterproof and it helps protect the deeper structures. The cells in the basal layer are mostly what we call keratocytes, while 5–10 percent are pigmented cells called melanocytes.

Skin cancer is the development of malignant change in the cells of this basal layer and can be any of the common forms of skin cancer.

- basal cell cancer (BCC)
- squamous cell cancer (SCC)
- malignant melanoma

Malignant change means the cells develop the ability to grow in an uncontrolled manner, and in some cases can spread throughout the body. More than 90 percent of cases are caused by ultraviolet (UV) radiation from the sun.

Basal Cell Cancer and Squamous Cell Cancer of the Skin

Basal cell cancer (BCC) and squamous cell cancer (SCC) of the skin are often grouped together as nonmelanoma skin cancer. BCCs are more common, accounting for 80 percent of nonmelanoma skin cancers. While SCC and BCC might look and behave differently, they have a common origin in the nonpigmented cells of the basal layer of the skin.

Long-term UV radiation can damage the DNA in these cells, so they are more prone to become malignant. Unlike melanoma, which seems to be stimulated by intermittent skin burning and can occur anywhere in the body, nonmelanoma skin cancers occur in the sun-exposed areas themselves. They are most common on the face, head, neck, limbs, and also on the trunk of the body in people who do not regularly wear shirts when in the sun. Not surprisingly, they are more common on the side closest to the window in people who do a lot of driving.

SCC skin cancers generally look different than BCCs in that they often have a layer of keratin on their surface, and this makes them feel rough to the touch. Keratin is a protein made by the keratinocytes and its function is to anchor the cells together. In SCC, this becomes heaped up in a thick layer.

A similar and more common condition in which the keratin becomes heaped up in patches on the skin is solar keratosis, also known as actinic keratosis. While this is benign, it is regarded as a precursor to SCC, as it not uncommonly progresses to SCC. It can therefore be regarded as a premalignant condition so by treating this, SCC might be prevented.

BCC skin cancers generally do not have the keratin build-up that characterizes SCC. They usually appear as a clump of tiny white nodules, often described as "pearls," and sometimes with an ulcer in the center of this cluster of "pearls." While they are more common in people with solar keratoses, the solar keratoses are more an indication that this is an area of severely sun-damaged skin, rather than the precursor of the BCC.

The big difference between and SCCs and BCCs, and also melanoma, is the frequency with which they metastasize. With metastasis, bits break off from the cancer and travel around the body, lodge and grow elsewhere, and become a life-threatening situation. With BCC, this almost never happens; with SCC, it occasionally happens; and with malignant melanoma, it is relatively common.

Malignant Melanoma

Scattered among the basal cells that are constantly regenerating the skin and forming roughly 5–10 percent of the cells in this layer, are pigment cells. These are called melanocytes and they form melanin, a dark substance that absorbs ultraviolet B (UVB) radiation from the sun and helps protect us from harmful effects of UVB.

The amount of melanin in the cells varies, both with genetics and with sunlight. For example, our skin gets darker as we tan after exposure to sunlight, and this is the cells producing more melanin to protect us from the increased exposure. Naturally dark-skinned races have the same proportion of melanocytes in their skin, but they have a much higher concentration of melanin in these cells.

When the melanocytes undergo malignant change, they form the cancer known as malignant melanoma, often shortened to melanoma. The cells proliferate in an uncontrolled growth, forming a dark lump or mark on the skin, and eventually bits break off and travel along lymphatics or in the blood and lodge in other parts of the body as metastases.

While melanoma occurs mostly in sun-exposed parts of the body, it can occur in other sites that do not get sun exposure. It can also occur in some unusual sites such as under the nails, on the palms of the hands, on the soles of the feet, and in the eye.

Some melanomas are not pigmented, being pale, rather than dark, and this makes diagnosis difficult. As with many cancers, it also occurs in a noninvasive form called in situ melanoma. While this cannot spread, it is common for invasive melanoma to form within this area, so removal of in situ melanoma is an important way of preventing malignant melanoma.

Who Gets Skin Cancer?

SCC and BCC skin cancers are predominantly caused by UVB radiation by a direct action on the DNA in the skin, although UVA is also important. For melanoma, UVA is more important, with the UVA resulting in the release of free radicals that in turn damage DNA. Reducing UV radiation is the most effective means of preventing these cancers. DNA damage is cumulative, with the more exposure over a lifetime, the greater the damage. The skin of young people is particularly sensitive to this UV damage.

The incidence of all types of skin cancer has increased over the last couple of decades. In the UK, overall the rate of melanoma has doubled since the 1990s, although it has reduced in people under 40. Similarly, the incidence of SCC of the skin has also increased. The most likely reason melanoma is decreasing in younger people is education about the harm of excess sun exposure, so this group now is more likely to cover-up and use sunscreens. For the older population, it is likely that their behavior when younger is catching up with them, such as spending more time in the sun with less covering of clothing, and the use of tanning beds.

Another reason for the increase in skin cancers relates to the increase in people who are overweight or obese, as excess body fat increases skin cancer risk. This is reversible, for compared to obese people who do not lose weight, weight-loss surgery results in a more than a 60 percent reduction in the chances of developing malignant melanoma.

The likelihood of skin cancer developing include the following factors.

Skin Color

The likelihood of developing skin cancer is largely determined by natural skin color, although sun exposure also plays an important part. The people most at risk are pale-skinned, freckled redheads who burn easily, such as those of Celtic origin, while it is rare among races who have naturally dark-pigmented skin, such as those of African Negroid origin.

Races with intermediate levels of skin pigmentation have intermediate risk. For example, in the US, the incidence of developing melanoma per 100,000 individuals each year is 27.2 for white-skinned people, 4.5 for Hispanics, 1.7 for Asians, and 1.1 for black-skinned people. The same principle applies to nonmelanoma skin cancers. For white-skinned people, the rate of SCC development is 150–350/100,000 population per year, the higher figure being for males. For dark-skinned individuals, it is only about 3 per 100,000, a hundredfold difference!

Where You Live

The likelihood of developing skin cancer is also determined by the intensity of the sunlight in your environment. The closer you live to the equator, the greater the risk. Queensland, Australia, a state situated in the tropics and populated mostly by white-skinned individuals, has the highest rate of melanoma in the world. For SCC, the incidence of the condition in Australian men is more than 1,000 per 100,000 population each year, while in Finland it is only 6 per 100,000.

How Much You Have Been Exposed to UV Radiation

UV exposure leads to skin cancer. The more UV exposure, the greater the risk. It is a little different for the various types of skin cancer. For SCC, it depends largely on the total lifetime exposure. One study suggested that the greatest risk came from over 30,000 hours of lifetime sun exposure. For BCC and melanoma, intermittent intense sun exposure seems to be more important, such as sunburn in childhood. Young people who have had five or more episodes of severe sunburn during their life double their chances of getting a melanoma.

The sun is not the only source of UV radiation. Studies show that tanning beds result in a significantly increased risk of developing all forms of skin cancer. For SCC, the risk is about a 65 percent increase, but for melanoma, it is much higher. Use of a tanning bed results in between a doubling and sixfold increase in the risk of developing melanoma. This has led to many countries either banning, or restricting access to, tanning salons.

Age of UV Exposure

For melanoma and also for basal cell cancer, UV exposure during childhood and adolescence is particularly harmful. For squamous cell cancer, it seems to be more the accumulated exposure over a lifetime.

Moles

Some people naturally have a lot of moles. The medical term for moles is naevi, and these are not to be confused with freckles. Having multiple moles predisposes to melanoma, with 20–30 percent of melanomas arising in moles.

This does mean that 70–80 percent of melanomas do not arise in pre-existing moles, so just because you do not have many moles, does not mean you cannot get melanoma.

The more moles you have, the higher the risk of getting melanoma. People with 50–100 moles have about a twentyfold increased risk compared to people with low mole counts. Even people with twenty-five moles have a slightly increased risk. Anyone with a lot of moles should have regular skin checks, and whole-body photography is a good idea to help monitor changes. Any moles that have changed should be removed.

Immunosuppression

Another condition that predisposes people to skin cancer is immunosuppression. The most common situation where this occurs is after organ transplant, where the immune system needs to be suppressed by drugs so the kidney, liver, or other organ that has been transplanted is not rejected. Other situations of immunosuppression include some lymphoma patients and in people with HIV infection.

Studies of organ-transplant patients show that they have more than three times the chance of developing melanoma, and an up to 250-fold increase for SCC, compared to people who have not had a transplant. The longer the duration of immunosuppression and the greater the sunlight exposure in these people, the greater the risk. In Australia, 45 percent of transplant patients will develop an SCC after ten years, compared to only 10–15 percent of transplant patients in Europe. Furthermore, when an SCC develops in an immunosuppressed patient, it tends to be more aggressive.

Genetics

About 10 percent of melanomas occur in someone who has a strong family history of melanoma. For SCC, a family history of SCC results in a doubling of risk. When studying family history and a disease such as skin cancer, it can be difficult to separate familial behavioral patterns, such as sunbathing, from an inherited predisposition. Nevertheless, it is likely that there are inherited genes that predispose to skin cancer.

Preventing Skin Cancer

Clearly you cannot change your racial origin and skin color, so you have to look after the skin with which you were born. It is impractical for most people to move to a higher latitude where the sun is not only less intense, but the cooler climate provides more incentive to cover the body with clothes.

The best thing to do is to just avoid intensive sunlight. Do this by minimizing the time spent outside in the middle of the day when the sun is most intense and wear sun-protective clothing, such as a hat and long sleeves. If it is necessary to go out during times of intense sunlight, exposed skin should be covered with a high sun protection factor (SPF) sun-blocking cream. This is most important in adolescents and children, in whom exposure is believed to do the most damage.

Preventing UV Exposure

Preventing UV radiation exposure is the most important thing you can do to prevent skin cancer. This is not difficult, but it does require some dedication. It is too easy to say, "I'm just going out for a few minutes" and not put on sunscreen, then end up spending long enough in the sun to get significant exposure. Part of the problem is not knowing how much UV exposure is good and how much is bad.

Exposure to some sunshine is important for our general health. Sunshine is the most important source of vitamin D, and it is essential for bone health. It can also prevent depression and helps prevent multiple sclerosis. It has been estimated that when the UV index is three or above, you get enough vitamin D by spending a few minutes outside each day. To get adequate vitamin D in winter or in high latitudes when the UV index is often below three, you need to spend longer outside, preferably in the middle of the day with skin exposed.

There are multiple ways to help prevent excessive exposure to UV radiation. This is particularly important at times when there is a high UV index or when surrounded by water or snow, as these reflect UV and so increase the intensity of exposure. The UV index for any particular time of day and location is readily available on most weather apps. If the UV index is above three, take sun-protective action.

Clothing

Choose sun-protective clothing.

- Wear long-sleeved clothing, preferably with a high neck. Cover legs.
- Choose a tight weave, so there are no gaps to let light through.
- Dark-colored materials absorb more UV so less reaches the skin.
- Synthetics are better than cotton, largely because they are generally elastic and have fewer holes to let light through, but also because they are often shiny and reflect light. For example, light white cotton material has an SPF of 5, so it lets through one-fifth sunlight, while Lycra and elastic materials have an SPF of 50, so they let through one-fiftieth sunlight.

Hats and Sunglasses

To be effective, hats need to be wide-brimmed and with a tight weave, preferably made of a synthetic material. Sunglasses generally block 99–100 percent of both UVA and UVB and are needed not just for eye protection; skin cancers can form on the eyelids. Preferably they should be the wraparound type. Schools in Australia have a "no hat, no play" policy, so children who don't wear a hat are not permitted outside during breaks.

Sunscreen

Sunscreens are measured by their SPF factor and this is a measure of UVB protection. A rough guide is that if it takes fifteen minutes to burn your skin, an SPF 15 sunscreen properly applied will take fifteen times longer to burn, about 3.5 hours. Use an SPF 30 cream, or higher, and remember that no sunscreen is 100 percent effective!

Sunscreens usually contain a number of ingredients that prevent UV from reaching the skin. These are either chemicals that absorb UV, or substances that form a physical barrier to UV, such as microfine or even nanosized particles of zinc or titanium. The nano preparations are so fine, they are virtually clear.

There has been some concern that nanoparticles get into the blood, but this is not true—they do not get through all the layers of the skin, staying in the outer layers of the skin. While the SPF on the label is a measure of its effectiveness at blocking UVB, ideally, it should also block UVA. These are often referred to as broad-spectrum sun creams. Do your internet research before making your purchase. Get a broad-spectrum cream.

A common mistake is to not apply enough sunscreen. It is recommended you use a teaspoon for the face and neck, a teaspoon for each arm and each leg, and a teaspoon each for trunk front and back. It should be applied twenty minutes before going out, as it takes some time to bind to the skin and be effective. It should be reapplied every two hours, as this is about the time it takes for it to be rubbed or sweated off.

Research has shown that using sunscreens does help reduce skin cancers. In an Australian trial, 1,621 people were randomly allocated to either "active use" where SPF 15+ cream was freely available and use encouraged, or "passive use" where the participants supplied their own cream and used it at their discretion.

After ten years of follow-up, only three invasive melanomas had developed in the active group compared to eleven in the passive group, a 75 percent reduction. Similarly, there was a 40 percent reduction in the development of SCCs, and a 50 percent reduction in noninvasive melanoma. Studies have also shown there is a reduction in the number of moles that develop in children who use sunscreens.

Car Windows

Spending a lot of time in a car is a source of significant sun exposure. The front windshield is, by law, made from laminated glass. This means there are two layers of glass with a layer of plastic sandwiched between them. While the aim is to reduce injury in the event of a crash, it also reduces UV exposure, as the plastic absorbs virtually all of UVA and UVB, giving it an SPF of 50 or more.

The side windows in most cars are different and are made of a single layer of glass. This blocks out virtually all UVB, but the glass lets through 80 percent of UVA. It does depend on the car manufacturer as some use high-SPF glass for the side windows too. To be safe, use a sunscreen for long trips.

Tanning

Multiple studies have shown that indoor tanning beds significantly increase a person's chances of developing both melanoma and nonmelanoma skin cancers. They are to be avoided. If a tan is required, fake tanning lotions have been shown to be harmless.

Treat Sun-Damaged Skin

Many people reach adulthood not realizing they have spent too much time in the sun in their youth. They then find they are developing actinic keratoses, a precancer feature of sun damage, or even skin cancers. The damage done can be reversed to some extent by topical treatments. By doing this, the rate at which new skin cancers develop is slowed, and in particular, surgery for skin cancers can be avoided. It can save pain, disfigurement, and cost.

There are two groups of these skin creams. One is 5 Fluorouracil (5FU) cream, which is a topical chemotherapy where the 5FU kills cancer cells in the skin before they become apparent as a lump or ulcer. The other type of cream stimulates the body's own immune system to fight the cancer cells hidden in the skin, so it has the same effect. It is a type of immunotherapy, with the most common drug of this type called imiquimod. The immune therapy seems a more natural approach, using the body's own defense system, rather than chemotherapy. These treatments are also effective for established skin cancers when small.

In one study, 932 US veterans who had at least three skin cancers treated in the last five years were randomly allocated to have either a 5FU cream treatment twice daily to their face and ears for two to four weeks or a placebo cream. Both groups also received SPF 30+ cream and were advised how to use it. They were followed for up to four years to determine how many new skin cancers they developed on their face and ears.

In the 5FU cream group, there was a 75 percent reduction in the number of SCCs that developed in the first year, and an 11 percent reduction in the number of BCCs. The treatment group had significantly less skin cancer surgery than the placebo group. The benefit, however, was not maintained for the full four years, and it became apparent that the treatment needs to be reapplied every year or two.

When applied for the first time, with both forms of treatment, most people get a marked reaction with redness and sometimes weeping of the skin. Once the treatment is completed in a few weeks, a dry scab forms that falls off and reveals the healthy skin underneath. The reaction is due to the body's inflammatory reaction that it mounts to deal with the dead cancer cells that are now present in the skin. It is not an allergy to the chemical.

Because of this reaction, it is sensible to treat the affected area a bit at a time. For subsequent treatments, the reaction is generally not so intense, as the number of dead cells to be dealt with is less. Interestingly, when using the immunotherapy type of creams, subsequent treatments result in a much earlier reaction, as the body's immune system has a memory and works faster.

Vitamin B3

Taking the form of vitamin B3 known as nicotinamide has been shown to reduce the chances of developing nonmelanoma skin cancer. In a clinical trial, 400 people who had previously been treated for at least two nonmelanoma skin cancers were enrolled, with half taking oral vitamin B3, 500 mg twice a day, and the others taking a placebo. After twelve months, those who took the vitamin B3 had a lower chance of getting either a new BCC or SCC. For SCC, there was a 30 percent reduction, a bit less for BCCs. For something that is side-effect free and as harmless as B3, this is a remarkable result.

Taking B3 should be seriously considered by anyone who is prone to developing skin cancers. Once the trial had finished after twelve months and the B3 stopped, the benefit did not continue, which means this is something you need to continue taking. There are several forms of vitamin B3 and it is important that the nicotinamide form be taken, not other forms such as niacin or nicotinic acid. Nicotinamide is believed to work by enhancing the DNA repair after damage by UV radiation, and it also reduces the level of immune suppression brought on by UV radiation.

Excess Body Fat

Obesity significantly increases the chances of getting a number of cancers, including skin cancers. What was not certain until recently was whether losing excess weight reversed this risk. A study of more than 4,000 obese people in Sweden has shown that weight loss does reverse this risk. Half had obesity surgery and had a long-term weight loss of about 20 kg (44 lb), while the others did not have surgery and did not lose significant weight.

The groups were followed for eighteen years and the numbers of cancers subsequently developed in each group has been compared. Those in the obesity surgery group developed twenty-three skin cancers while the others got forty-one, a more than 40 percent reduction.

With melanoma, this reduction in risk was even higher, with twelve melanomas in the weight-loss group compared to twenty-nine in the other. This is a more than a 60 percent reduction. For people who are overweight, it is possible to significantly reduce your skin cancer risk by losing weight.

Retinoids

Retinoids are chemically related to vitamin A and are thought to be important as a regulator of cell proliferation and as activator of tumor-suppressor genes. They can be given by mouth or applied to the skin as a lotion. They have been studied widely in regard to their ability to reverse solar damage of the skin and in particular prevent skin cancers.

While some studies have not been convincing about benefit, most do show that the oral forms reduce the number of SCCs that develop in sun-damaged skin. In one trial, over 2,000 people with sun-damaged skin were randomly allocated to either take 25,000 units of retinol by mouth daily or a placebo. Those taking retinol had a 25 percent reduction in the number of new skin SCCs they developed. However, those taking retinol did have a rise in their triglyceride and cholesterol levels, so it might increase the risk of heart disease.

To Prevent Skin Cancer

If Your Skin Is Not Sun-Damaged, Keep It That Way

- Wear sun-protective clothing, hats, and sunglasses.
- Use SPF 30+ or higher sunscreen cream if going out when the UV index is above three.

If You Already Have Sun-Damaged Skin

- Prevent further damage by sun-protective clothing and SPF 30+ cream.
- Take vitamin B3 500 mg twice daily.
- Consider treating the more severely damaged areas with a course of imiquimod or 5FU cream and repeat every few years.
- If you have had a skin cancer, especially melanoma, and you are overweight, try to lose the excess fat.

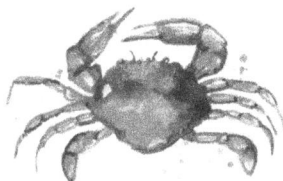

Thyroid Cancer

What Is Thyroid Cancer?

Thyroid cancer is not common and when it does occur, treatment is by surgery and high-dose radioactive iodine. For most forms of thyroid cancer, this is nearly always curative. It is usually detected as a lump in the front of the neck.

Who Gets Thyroid Cancer?

This type of cancer occurs more often in younger people. Exposure of the neck to radiation in childhood increases thyroid cancer risk. Because this is well-known, neck radiation in childhood and young adults is avoided as much as possible. One situation where it might occur is during radiation treatment of a childhood cancer. When this is necessary, or even during a CT scan of adjacent areas done for diagnostic purposes, a lead shield is used to protect the neck.

Another circumstance where there might be thyroid radiation in childhood is after a nuclear accident such as those in Chernobyl and Fukushima. Radioactive nuclear waste in the form of radioactive iodine (I-131) can be taken up by the body. Iodine is naturally concentrated in the thyroid gland to make thyroxine and the body cannot distinguish between normal and radioactive iodine. The thyroid is thus exposed to radiation, predisposing it to cancer. Fortunately, nuclear accidents are rare and atmospheric nuclear bomb testing no longer takes place.

Preventing Thyroid Cancer

People who have excess body fat have an almost 20 percent increased risk of getting thyroid cancer, and this is particularly so for obese people.

Avoid radiation of any kind for children, unless absolutely necessary. This includes being sure that appropriate shields are used during medical visits and dental visits. Dental assistants should use a lead apron that covers the neck when taking X-rays of the teeth and mouth.

To Prevent Thyroid Cancer

- Avoid preventable radiation, such as a neck CT scan
- Be sure that appropriate shields are used when X-rays are done.
- Lose excess body fat.

Brain Tumors

What Are Brain Tumors?

Most primary brain tumors are either benign meningiomas, the meninges being the layer of tissue that lines the brain, or a variety of glial tumors of the brain cells. Gliomas vary from low-grade, slow-growing malignant tumors to high-grade, fast-growing cancers, such as the glioblastoma. Most people first notice a headache, but other features include seizures or loss of function of part of the body. They are diagnosed by brain CT or MRI scans.

Who Gets Brain Tumors?

This type of cancer is more common in children and older adults. Men are more likely to develop a brain tumor than women. Over the last fifteen years, the frequency with which brain tumors occur has steadily decreased. There is a higher rate of incidence for some workers in specialized industries, such as agricultural workers, where there is exposure to chemicals.

Preventing Brain Tumors

Ionizing Radiation

Ionizing radiation is a well-recognized cause of brain cancer, especially in children, so exposure of the brain to radiation should be kept to a minimum. As with thyroid cancer, the most common radiation reason is the treatment of a childhood cancer by radiation therapy. In particular, brain irradiation as part of childhood leukemia treatment means that survivors have an increased risk of developing a brain tumor later in life.

As many as 15 percent of children who have brain irradiation will develop a brain tumor many years later, and especially so if they had the irradiation before the age of five. Childhood brain irradiation from diagnostic CT scans also increases risk, as does exposure to nuclear waste.

Herbicides and Pesticides

Agricultural workers, and others who might be exposed to herbicides and pesticides, are at a slightly higher risk of developing brain tumors.

Allergies

People with allergies, such as asthma, eczema, and hay fever, have a significantly lower risk of developing brain tumors. A high immunoglobulin E (IgE) level in the blood, an immune protein, is associated with reduced brain tumor risk. These findings suggest the body's immune system plays an important part in controlling brain tumor development.

Electromagnetic and Radiofrequency Radiation

Exposure to electromagnetic radiation, such as living close to overhead power lines or even from the electrical wiring in the roof of a house and radiofrequency radiation, such as from cell phones, have not been shown to cause brain tumors. Considering the widespread use of cell phones, one would expect the incidence of brain tumors to be rising. In fact, the opposite is the case, with a gradual reduction in incidence.

To Prevent Brain Tumors

- Avoid preventable radiation, such as a brain CT scan.
- Avoid pesticides and herbicides,

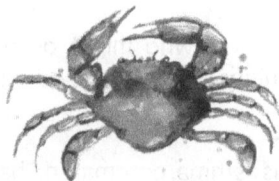

Blood and Lymphatic Cancers

What Are Blood and Lymphatic Cancers?

Cancers of the blood and lymphatic tissues are part of a group of tumors called hemopoietic neoplasms. These include lymphomas and leukemias, and there are dozens of subtypes.

Hodgkin's lymphoma accounts for about 10 percent of these cancers and mostly occur in young adults. It makes itself apparent by an enlarged lymph node, and treatment is usually curative.

Non-Hodgkin's lymphoma is much less common in young adults, but when it occurs it can be an aggressive disease, while in older adults it is usually slower growing. As with Hodgkin's lymphoma, lymph-node enlargement is most common, but it can present in a variety of other ways.

There are four main groups of leukemias: acute lymphoblastic, acute myeloid, chronic lymphocytic, and chronic myeloid. There are also less-common types.

Preventing Blood and Lymphatic Cancers

Viral Infections

There is an increased risk of Hodgkin's lymphoma in people with a past infection with the infectious mononucleosis virus (EBV). Other viral infections, such as measles, mumps, chickenpox, and whooping cough, seem to have a protective effect for Hodgkin's lymphoma.

Immunosuppression

People taking immunosuppressive drugs, such as those who have had a transplant, are at higher risk for lymphomas. Other immunosuppression, such as HIV, or autoimmune diseases, such as rheumatoid arthritis or systemic lupus, is also associated with an increased risk of developing lymphoma.

Pesticides

Exposure to organophosphate pesticides has been shown to increase the risk of developing non-Hodgkin's lymphoma and leukemia. A study of 155,000 farmers found those with exposure to pesticides had double the risk of developing non-Hodgkin's lymphoma, and the risk increased with the number of acres sprayed. People who eat predominantly organic foods have a lower incidence of non-Hodgkin's lymphoma.

Ionizing Radiation

Ionizing radiation is a well-recognized cause of leukemia, as first seen in survivors of the atomic bombs dropped on Hiroshima and Nagasaki.

Excess Body Fat

Obesity is associated with an increased risk of non-Hodgkin's lymphoma, also multiple myeloma, another form of hemopoietic cancer.

Breast Prostheses

Although rare, breast implant-associated anaplastic large cell lymphoma (BIA-ALCL) needs to be mentioned, because it is a preventable form of cancer. It can develop in the fibrous tissue that forms around a breast implant. The frequency is uncertain, as different studies have come up with different statistics, but it occurs in between 1 in 4,000 and 1 in 30,000 women who have long-standing breast implants. It occurs most commonly with textured prostheses but can also occur a with smooth-surfaced breast prosthesis.

To Prevent Blood and Lymphatic Cancers

- Avoid unnecessary radiation.
- Avoid pesticides and herbicides.
- Lose excess body fat

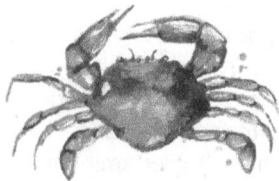

The Final Word

The final word is that the decision is yours. Do you really want to do everything you can to reduce your chances of getting cancer? Are you prepared to make the hard decisions to change your lifestyle to one that minimizes cancer risk?

Lifestyle changes can be hard. The things you can change and that have the greatest impact for preventing cancer are these lifestyle recommendations that you control.

- Eat a healthy diet. (up to 30 percent)
- Do not use tobacco. (19 percent)
- Treat or vaccinate for cancer-causing infections. (17 percent)
- Lose excess body fat. (8 percent)
- Limit alcohol consumption. (6 percent)
- Avoid UV radiation. (5 percent)
- Be physically active. (3 percent)
- Drink coffee.
- Limit unnecessary diagnostic tests that involve high doses of radiation, such as CT or PET scans.

The percent figures in parentheses indicate how much each of these factors contributes to cancer worldwide, and could be prevented by changes that you make to your lifestyle. Some are inter-related, such as eating a healthy diet and losing excess body fat, so these contributions cannot be totaled.

Diet

A diet consisting of mainly fruits and vegetables, whole grains, dairy products, and fish; and with limited red meat, processed and pickled foods, and highly refined foods, will significantly reduce cancer risk. If you can, choose organic foods and reduce pesticide exposure. For vegans or people with lactose intolerance, take calcium supplements.

Tobacco Use

Stopping smoking is difficult, but this is the biggest single cause of cancer and the biggest killer.

Vaccination and Treating Chronic Infections

Widespread vaccination has the possibility of nearly eliminating hepatitis B and HPV infections. Hepatitis C and *Helicobacter pylori* infections are treatable. By doing these things, most liver, many gastric, and nearly all cervical cancers could be prevented.

Lose Excess Fat

Excess fat is an important cause of many cancers. Weight loss is difficult but definitely worthwhile from a cancer point-of-view.

Alcohol Consumption

Anything more than light drinking is a significant cause of cancer and should be avoided.

UV Radiation

Preventing excess UV radiation is simple and can prevent skin cancers. Remember that some sun exposure is important for vitamin D production.

Physical Activity

Being physically active plays a small but important part in cancer prevention.

Drinking Coffee

Coffee drinking can help prevent some cancers, especially biliary and liver cancers.

Limit Unnecessary Diagnostic X-Rays

Tests that involve high doses of radiation, such as chest and abdominal CT or PET scans, have the potential to damage DNA and so should only be undertaken if there is a good medical indication. This is especially so in children or if they are being repeated on multiple occasions.

Cancer can be a dreadful disease. Prevention is by far the best and worth the challenge to make a change.

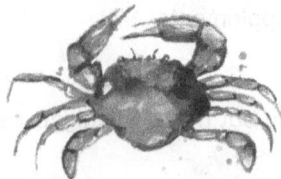

Glossary of Terms

ACTH - Adrenocorticotrophic hormone, released from the pituitary gland in response to stress.

Adenomatous polyps - Outgrowth from the wall of the bowel that has the potential to become a bowel cancer.

Adrenaline - A hormone produced by the adrenal gland in response to stimuli, such as stress or physical activity.

Antioxidant - A chemical that prevents oxidation and so free radicals.

Antiproliferative - The process of prevention of cell growth.

Apoptosis - The process by which the body controls cell death.

Atrophy - The wasting away of a body structure.

Bariatric surgery - An operation that encourages weight loss.

Bioactive - Something that can act on living tissue.

BRCA mutation - An inherited mutation of tumor-suppressor genes.

Carcinogen - A substance capable of causing cancer.

CHEK2 mutation - An inherited mutation of a tumor-suppressor gene.

Chemoprevention - A medication that can prevent a disease.

CIN - Cervical intraepithelial neoplasia is the precancerous transformation of cells on the cervix of the uterus.

Cortisol - A steroid hormone produced by the adrenal gland in response to stress.

Diuretic - A drug that results in urine production.

DNA - Two chains of elements that form a double helix and carry the genetic instructions.

Dopamine - A hormone that transmits instructions between nerves.

Dysplasia - Pathological term describing abnormal cellular growth.

Endometriosis - Growth of the uterine lining cells outside the uterus.

Endoscopy - Passage of a flexible fiberoptic tube to allow visualization of the inside of organs, usually stomach or colon.

Fallopian tube - Tubular structure attached to the uterus, which carries the egg from ovary to uterus prior to fertilization.

Germline mutation - Inherited abnormality of chromosomal DNA in sperm or ovum cells that allows transmission to offspring.

Hemopoietic - The body system that makes the blood elements.

Hyperplasia - An increase in cell proliferation.

IGF-1 - Hormone similar to insulin that promotes growth.

Ileostomy - Opening of small bowel onto skin, usually on the abdomen and requiring a bag to collect effluent.

Immune surveillance - Ability of the immune system to detect abnormalities.

Insulin resistance - A situation where cells fail to respond to the hormone insulin.

Keratin - A protein found in the skin that protects the skin cells. Hair and nails, also animal hooves and horns, are made of keratin.

Metastasis - The process of spread of cancer to distant parts of the body

Mitosis - Division of a cell into two daughter cells.

mSv - milliSievert, a measure of radiation dose.

Mutagenic - The effect of a chemical that changes DNA to increase the rate of mutations.

Nasopharynx - The airway passage situated just above the back of the mouth.

Neoplasm - Another name for a growth of cells, also known as a tumor.

Nuclear scan - Diagnostic test that uses the emissions from a radioactive isotope to provide an image of some body part.

Oestradiol - The main natural female sex hormone.

Oncogene - A gene that has the potential to cause cancer.

Oncovirus - A virus that has the potential to cause cancer.

Oral cavity - The structures surrounding the mouth.

Oropharynx - The passage situated at the back of the mouth through which passes air for breathing and ingested food.

Phytochemical - A chemical of plant origin.

Phytoestrogen - A plant chemical that has an estrogenic action.

Placebo - A substance that has no effect on the body.

Progesterone - A natural female sex hormone involved in the menstrual cycle and pregnancy.

Progestin - Synthetic female sex hormone related to progesterone.

Prolactin - Natural female hormone involved in milk production.

Renal tract - Urine excretion conduits including renal pelvis, ureter, bladder, and urethra.

Salpingo-oophorectomy - Operation to remove ovaries and Fallopian tubes

Serotonin - A hormone that facilitates information transmission between nerves, especially in the gut.

Somatic mutation - An abnormality of chromosomal DNA in a cell.

Stoma - Opening of bowel onto skin, usually on the abdomen and requiring a bag to collect effluent.

Telomere - Region at the end of a chromosome that protects it from deterioration, becoming shorter with age.

Tumor-suppressor gene - A gene that protects a cell from becoming cancer.

Urothelium - The lining layer of the renal tract.

Villous polyp - A colonic polyp that has a cauliflower-like appearance and has the potential to become a cancer.

Acknowledgments

I would like to thank my good friends, Linda and Faye, who took the time and had the patience to work through my first draft and provide such useful advice. I really do appreciate your help.

To my family members who helped review the manuscript, many thanks for their advice and corrections.

I would also like to thank Maggie Dent, who provided the encouragement that it was possible to write a book—she does not realize how often I looked to her books as a guide and inspiration. Thank you, Maggie, for giving them to me.

And to Alison Fennell, who, in the blink of an eye, produced such amazing artwork for the cover—thank you, Alison. I am forever indebted to you.

Many thanks also to Joni Wilson, who did a fantastic job of editing and providing helpful advice and guidance for this novice writer.

I must also thank Katharine Middleton of Ink Box Graphics who did such a great job setting out the book.

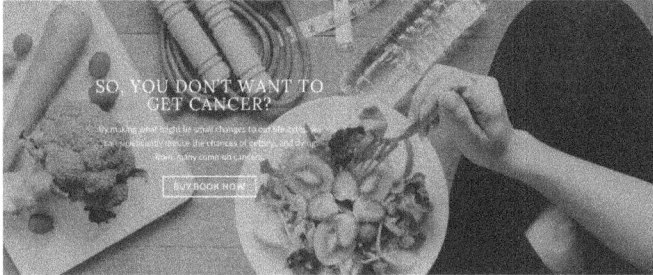

For cancer prevention articles, resources and newsletter sign-up visit:

www.dontwantcancer.com.au

'Cancer impacts families everywhere. Rather than just hope it doesn't arrive - we all need to know what are the things we can do to prevent getting it in the first place. Dr David Ingram has written a fascinating, comprehensive guide on how not to get cancer! So even if you don't worry about yourself - you need to get this book so you can help your kids and grandkids improve their chances not to get cancer - and you need to do it now!'

Maggie Dent - Author, Parenting and Resilience Educator.

"This is a concise and evidence-based must read for those of you wanting to know the truth about factors which increases risk of getting cancer and what you can do to minimise this risk."

Professor Arlene Chan - Medical Oncologist